Dinner Music

How to Compose the Permanently Perfect Diet

Dinner Music
How to Compose the Permanently Perfect Diet

Richard Donze

KROSHKA BOOKS
Commack, NY
1998

Editorial Production: Susan Boriotti
Office Manager: Annette Hellinger
Graphics: Frank Grucci and John T'Lustachowski
Information Editor: Tatiana Shohov
Book Production: Donna Dennis, Patrick Devin, Christinc Mathosian, Tammy
            Sauter and Diane Sharp
Circulation: Maryanne Schmidt
Marketing/Sales: Cathy DeGregory

Library of Congress Cataloging-in-Publication Data

Donze, Richard.
Dinner Music : how to compose the permanently perfect diet /
Richard Donze.
    p.   cm.
   ISBN 1-56072-508-7
   1. Nutrition.   2. Health I. Title.
RA784.D66   1997   97-41665
613.2—dc21   CIP

The authors and publisher haven taken care in preparation of this book, but make no
expressed or implied warranty of any kind and assume no responsibility for any errors
or omissions. No liability is assumed for incidental or consequential damages in
connection with or arising out of information contained in this book.

This publication is designed to provide accurate and authoritative information with
regard to the subject matter covered herein. It is sold with the clear understanding that
the publisher is not engaged in rendering legal or any other professional services. If
legal or any other expert assistance is required, the services of a competent person
should be sought. FROM A DECLARATION OF PARTICIPANTS JOINTLY
ADOPTED BY A COMMITTEE OF THE AMERICAN BAR ASSOCIATION AND
A COMMITTEE OF PUBLISHERS.

Printed in the United States of America

For Lucy, Kitty, and Sally Hope, who season the wood, provide the spark, and tend the flame

CONTENTS

Acknowledgements

This song has spilled out of the top of my head, an overflow of everything I have ever read, heard, or thought about eating and food. When I sing it I hear my own voice, but can also recognize other influences, threads of tune-ideas from other great nutrition composers. I owe a huge debt of gratitude to Anthony Sattilaro, MD, Michio Kushi, Nathan Pritikin, Michael Jacobson, PhD, William Castelli, MD, AnneMarie Colbin, Herman Aihara, Rudolph Ballentine, MD, and Michel Abehserrah. I am certain that many of their ideas have come out of me re-packaged and re-formulated, with a slightly different spin perhaps, but hopefully fresh.

I also want to thank Frank and Nadya Columbus at Kroshka Books. Like their namesake, they refused to believe that the nutrition world was flat, so they took a chance and sailed for the New World of food inspiration, in a different brain hemisphere.

I thank John Brown, my perennial writing teacher, who introduced me to John Donne's notion that "Words are our subtlest and delicatest outward creatures, being composed of thought and breath." On that line I also thank Charlene Breedlove, my poetry editor at JAMA, who has always encouraged me. I believe there is a poetic tone in this book which John and Charlene helped hone.

I thank my family and friends, the people who believe in me and supported me and eaten the whole grain-bean-vegetable experiments I've boiled, baked, steamed these last twenty years. Parents Sam and Lucy gave me life, love and unbounded confidence and optimism, Siblings Bob, George, and Rose (and their significant others Deb, Jane, and Frank) listened to my ideas, made suggestions, and Rose especially with her copy-writing expertise kept me focusing me on the ways to clarify what I was trying to say ("Bring this up, move it to the beginning, tell the reader what's in it for them"). Friends Jim (whom we all call "Brother") and Carol traveled with us to Maine and countless other closer places for something good to eat.

Daughters Elizabeth and Sarah are my ultimate inspiration. They are like two more parents, 180-degrees away from the first set, who also love and approve unconditionally and believe Dad can do anything. They also love my baked tofu.

Finally, I thank my wife Kathy who lived with and suffered through every dietary experiment. Over twenty years of marriage and nineteen years of medical practice I talked about "the book", and she kept me faithful to the task by moving herself philosophically to Missouri and saying "Show me". Well, honey, here it is.

Richard Donze
West Chester, PA
January 25, 1998

ABOUT THE AUTHOR

Dr. Richard Donze is a physician Board-Certified in Preventive Medicine and Family Practice. He has an undergraduate degree in English from the University of Pennsylvania, and received his medical degree from the Philadelphia College of Osteopathic Medicine. He also obtained a Master of Public Health post-doctoral degree from the Department of Preventive Medicine at the Medical College of Wisconsin.

Dr. Donze has integrated preventive medicine and nutritional counseling into his medical practice the past eighteen years. Between 1987 and 1989 he was a staff physician at the Pennsylvania Pritikin Center, a residential program for lifestyle modification. He has taught and lectured widely in medical school classes, continuing education conferences, at seminars sponsored by schools, service organizations, and local industries, and has been interviewed in the local media. He is currently the Corporate Vice-President for Medical Affairs at the Chester County Hospital in West Chester, Pennsylvania, while maintaining a limited practice with a hospital subsidiary.

Dr. Donze is also a published medical poet and essayist, and his work has appeared regularly in the *Journal of the American Medical Association,* as well as in other medical and lay publications. He lives in southeastern Pennsylvania with his wife and two children.

DISCLAIMERS

While the vignettes in this book are based upon actual experiences from my practice or amalgams of what I've seen and heard, all names of patients and clients are fictitious.

No part of this book is intended as medical advice. Anyone with a specific medical problem should consult a physician about appropriate treatment.

INTRODUCTION

This will be the most unusual and effective diet book you'll ever read because

- I've aimed it at the right side of your brain:
- there are no charts, graphs, or tables;
- there are no terrifying pictures or descriptions of clogged arteries;
- there are no promises of immortality;
- I won't tell you to weigh foods or balance amino acids;
- I won't tell you to bring a calculator to the market;
- I won't tell you to check the clock to see if it's time to eat fruit;
- there are no pyramids or other ancient stony wonders;
- there are no food lists with good and bad columns;
- there isn't a single recipe;
- nothing is for sale except ideas.

Instead I'll build you a bridge to span the brain-behavior gap, to get you from intellect and desire on one side to an appropriate diet on the other.

I've counseled thousands of people about diet and health during my eighteen years as a Preventive Medicine physician. When I advised my patients in 1979 to avoid fat, sugar, and processed foods and eat more whole grains, beans, vegetables and fruits for better health, many found these ideas relatively new. Now I see more people who know what to do and why to do it before they see me, aware that their diet-related obesity, high blood pressure, high cholesterol, and diabetes push them toward our three leading killers -

Heart Disease, Cancer, and Stroke. I attribute this change to more and better education in nutritionists' offices, hospital and health club seminars, and by groups such as the Center for Science in the Public Interest, the National Cholesterol Education Program, and the American Cancer Society. Our popular culture has also been inundated by diet-related books, magazine articles, talk-show interviews, five-minute local news health checks, TV doctor special reports, and insanity-stopping speeches.

Still I see people every day who are bedeviled by their diets, frustrated that they can't translate knowledge, need, and desire into action. They can chant familiar mantras about foolish fat and forgiving fiber, or say that white is out, as in rice and iceberg lettuce, while brown and dark green are in (whole grain and romaine). We can agree on sensible, attainable diet and health goals - no snacks or desserts till the weight is here or the cholesterol there. They can promise passionately to start on Monday, or as soon as they return from vacation, or definitely right after the New Year. But then so many fall short, or succeed for weeks or months only to slide back. They're like athletes who've sat in the locker room, stared at the X's and O's on the chalkboard, memorized the plays, and listened to the pep talks, but then can't execute on the field or court or rink.

When I had the same trouble, I thought the solution was to read a new book, take another course, and listen more intently to all the talk-shows and interviews, but I found myself reading, hearing and re-learning the same material. That's when I realized I was feeding the wrong side of my brain. My left half - the analytic, intellectual, data-loving side - already knew the facts, figures, milligrams, and percentages. I didn't execute appropriately and consistently until I involved my right brain - the artistic, intuitive, creative side.

I began to think less about fat grams, calories, and formal behavior modification techniques, and instead to create images, stories, analogies, and metaphors to attach to my diet. I took all those dry, sterile nutritional and psychological principles I'd read and heard and wove them into a fabric, an integrated right-brain permanent eating fix. It's not a scientifically tested method, model, or plan, but an anecdote. It's a song sung by a Preventive Medicine physician who has practiced long enough to recognize what works and what doesn't. I've found it so refreshing and effective for me that I am confident it can help you, too.

Let's move on, put this diet business behind us, fix our pounds-problem and attend to weightier issues. As a nation and a planet we have bigger fish to fry (or broil, as the case may be). Let's stop reading diet books (after you finish this one, of course) which invade more bookstore shelves every day, and re-discover poetry and novels.

Sit down now and take a few deep breaths. I'm going to share some images and ideas on the following pages which have helped me. Let them slide effortlessly into your right brain until they become your new programming. These diet cues will pop into your awareness without any need for you to summon them and direct your behavior automatically. You won't have to beat them into your head or pour over any material to memorize them for they are as easy to digest and absorb as the simple foods they will inspire you to eat.

If you're like a lot of my patients, you've been lost too long in the dark diet forest. If you can't find your way home even though you have the directions, perhaps it's because you always look left on your brain compass, seeing portion-sizes and milligram-heavy wrist-slapping rules, which can lead you down a frustratingly blind trail. I was lost, too, but found the way out. Fortunately, I marked the trail. Let me show you this new path, 180 degrees away, over on the right. Then watch yourself come into a clearing and look ahead. There's your diet home.

* * *

I've organized this book using the metaphor of a song and grouping the chapters into four sections. The first has chapters to generally orient you toward different ways of thinking about food and eating, as background or context. I call this the *Rhythm* section, since it's the rhythm that lays down the beat and gets you oriented to the song.

The chapters that mention actual foods or deal with food choices or selection I call *Melody*. Even though you need many components to make a whole song (or a whole diet), it's the melody that's most immediately recognizable, the part you identify as being the song, just as the actual food you select, put on your plate and in your mouth is what you recognize as your diet.

A few chapters address eating behavior, technique, and associated activities. I call these *Touch* because it's the fingers' touch on keys, strings, or valves or the lips' touch on a mouthpiece that helps produce the tone, the note. You can sit with an instrument and read the music, but no touch means no song. Behavior is like the touch for the diet, since you can know all the right ways to eat and have all the right foods in your cabinets, but still need the right touch to put it all together.

The final section is *Song*, with chapters that contain vignettes to show how I have attempted to combine rhythm, melody, and touch to create my dinner music, my eating song. Some of the meals I describe were planned while others just happened, but they should let you see how I have tried to walk the talk and play the tune the past eighteen years.

In a real song it all happens at once - touch, rhythm, melody - so to get that effect I mixed and scattered the chapters. This Introduction starts the rhythm, soon you'll hear some melody, and after that you're into the song. Feel free to tap your feet. Let the music rise, swirl around you, and carry you to your permanently perfect diet.

```
┌─────────────────┐
│   CHAPTER 1     │
└─────────────────┘
```

DISCIPLINE, TOOLS, AND A RIGHT BRAIN SONG

I want my patients to recognize the considerable discipline, will, and self-control they already possess. This is not some pop-psycho-babble affirmation, but a statement of fact. If you've ever tried to take control of your eating habits and temporarily failed, you may woefully claim you lack these character traits. I understand how you might reach this conclusion when you match what your head says you should have eaten with what ended up in your stomach. It must have been a breakdown in discipline, right? Not necessarily, because many times this assumption distorts the truth. I frequently observe that the real problem isn't a lack of will or self-control, but not having the correct tool. If you were unable to drive a nail with pliers, or loosen a bolt with a saw, you wouldn't say you lacked strength. Similarly, the patients I see often lack the correct diet tool, one that will let them demonstrate their will the way a hammer lets someone demonstrate nail-driving power. My missing diet tool was the right side of my brain.

I first learned the differences between the right and left brains in my medical school neuroanatomy class. I can visualize the slide projected onto the huge lecture hall screen showing which parts of the brain controlled specific muscle groups, glandular secretions, vision, and other bodily functions. The picture came alive when I was a junior student helping an intern and resident care for a man who'd had a stroke affecting his left brain circulation. Because language is controlled on the left side, he was unable to speak. His right brain was fine, though, so he could still sing.

I'm convinced that eating is a right brain song, but for years Western nutritional science has tried to assign this function to the left, reducing it to a simple matter of measuring and consuming nutrients such as protein, vitamins, and minerals. When I started to study nutrition in the late 1970's, I was the same way, stuffing my left brain with diet facts, figures, and plans, but it must have been the wrong tool because it didn't consistently lead me to eat better. The left brain proceeds too logically. It can decide in quiet moments that, yes, certainly, it would be a good idea to change the diet, lower the cholesterol, get more fiber and phytochemicals. It can tell you how many grams of fiber you need, because it read it or heard it and filed it away. It can calculate the calorie deficit you must generate to get off the excess poundage you want to lose before you start your vacation. It all sounds wonderful on the Sunday night before you start your Monday-diet. Then you go to work the next day, it's somebody's birthday, someone brings cake and, oh well, I guess you can start on Tuesday.

Where was the left brain when the cake came out? It had everything planned the night before. What went wrong? Many of the people I counsel believe they're just too weak and can't muster or sustain the force of will or discipline. So despite knowing what to do they fail and fail again to do it and get Monday's broken resolutions. They often end up whipping themselves and getting depressed about it, which unfortunately can lead to more dietary indiscretion, more frustration, more depression, and a perpetuating negative cycle.

To counter their distortions I tell my patients to focus on the things they do every day which require enormous amounts of will power and discipline. Just getting up in the morning - to go to work, or get the children fed and to the bus stop - requires will and discipline. I remind them that they might wake up and feel like skipping work, yet never do. But these same people can walk into the office or go to a party or a wedding and see something fatty or sweet or fatty and sweet they know they'd be better off without but still want, and indulge anyway. The urge to skip work lasts a minute or two, while the workday lasts eight hours. There's plenty of time to use will and discipline to overturn that simple, childlike desire. The yearning for the fatty-sweets is similarly short-lived, but the act is often over before the will and discipline have even been called to the scene.

Much of the conscious control over behavior lives in the left brain, and needs time to act, but unfortunately gets battled every day by impulsive desires which only take an instant to satisfy. Besides the impulses, though, the left brain has a hard time overturning our earliest dietary programming, everything we learned growing up about healthy eating. It was based on what we thought was true at the time - the righteousness of the four food groups, the importance of animal protein, the harmlessness of empty calories in a so-called balanced diet. In addition, food is so available in our culture with very few barriers to access. All someone needs to do to get a day's worth of fat calories is walk into a convenience store with a few dollars and buy a croissant-meat-cheese sandwich, a sugary beverage, and a shortening-plus-sugar cupcake or jumbo cookie. Finally, there's all the advertising, which is overtly or subliminally persuasive, promising popularity or fun beach parties for all those who eat or drink the correct soft drink.

Add them and you get our accumulated dietary experiences. Predictably, we learned to like certain things, and this affection was reinforced by the notion that it was good for us or at least not harmful. Just because we learn later that something we have grown to like is now considered bad for us, it may not be enough to negate the old program, especially when depression or some other emotional emptiness produces an overpowering hankering for pleasure or a sentimental attachment to a simpler, happier time. Patients often confide that they have certain comfort foods, items such as cake, candy, or ice cream which perhaps a mother or grandmother fed them as a child and which they still look for when their moods are low.

And because inappropriate eating behavior can happen automatically, there isn't enough time for any hope of influence by the plodding, linear left brain which has to look things up or retrieve information from storage.

My right brain images can act instantly, like Indiana Jones jumping on the horse to ride after the Ark while he shouts orders to his cohorts. He says, "I'm making it up as I go," but he's actually using his heroic, intuitive, split-second-deciding right brain. That type of behavior has to be cultivated, though, so let me plant thirty-or-so seeds in your right brain. They will sprout, grow, and save you when you're about to eat that donut someone brought to the office while your left brain methodically checks "D" for "donuts" but gets sidetracked when the file says it's under "P" for "pastry". Usually by the time your left brain figures out it was a bad idea to eat the lard-laden sugar-ring, it's already in, down the chute, digested, absorbed, and on its way to your abdomen or thighs. A properly programmed right brain will be your Indy, your whip-wielding hero, and snatch the poison from your hand before your hand gets to your mouth.

Thanks to all the books, talk-show interviews, magazine articles, info-mercials, and medical and nutritionist counseling, some re-programming is already underway. I recognize this whenever I discuss diet with patients and learn what they've read or heard and the changes they've made. Unfortunately, because so many people still have such a long way to go, it may not happen quickly enough for those who've already been wounded by their diets, so I want to speed up the process. All I ask from the people I counsel and from you is the courage, strength, and optimism to do it one more time. This will be the last time you have to do this, but it will feel like the clean-slate first time.

I frequently tell my patients to stop being so hard on themselves, to stop making themselves feel worse than they already do. They shouldn't confuse weakness or absence of will with simply lacking the appropriate equipment, or doom themselves by past mistakes. It's time to re-name failure and call it practice, then let it be the fertile soil for my image-seeds. I've watched will and discipline sprout and blossom where people thought they couldn't grow, and felt the power of self-control when the right tool-advice finally gets to the right side of the brain. I've heard the sound when the right brain works the diet. It's not the crash, thud, and metallic clang you hear when desire bangs against a left brain rule. It's a background hum, a purr of smooth mindful precision.

A permanently perfect diet is more than just knowing which foods to eat, just as beautiful music is more than knowing which notes to play. Both need the right brain to create the song.

CHAPTER 2

DINNER MUSIC

I imagine my food as music. I create a good meal, one that at the same time will satisfy and nourish without causing harm the way a composer or arranger creates a musical piece. I choose and blend the foods carefully, like instruments, depending on the sound, rhythm, and mood I want.

I listen to my patients' diets and often hear cacophony. They sound too loud in fat, sugar, salt, alcohol, and refined foods, and too soft in fiber, whole grains, beans, fresh vegetables, and fruits. I listen more closely with my stethoscope and hear the blood pressure pounding at 190. I read bad reviews on lab slips when the cholesterol or blood sugar is too high, and when these medical records go platinum, no one gets awards. My patients moan and wail while their melancholy families cover their ears, and it sounds like a dirge from the saddest opera.

Their attempts to fix things, the solutions they read about in diet books or hear about on TV, often seem misguided. They obsessively throw in the missing elements such as oat bran and wheat germ, because they eat too much refined white bread, rice, and pasta. They tear out the notorious poisons-du-jour, such as the way so many food producers have demonized fat lately, making sure that everything from snack crackers to ground turkey is as free of it as possible. If a little beta-carotene in a carrot is good, then a ton in a supplement must be better. Oat bran used to simply be part of oatmeal, beta-carotene a natural component of green and orange vegetables and fruits, and fat was fine and safe when it sat comfortably inside whole seeds and nuts. Let's start with these simple instruments, these basic foods such as whole grains, beans, fresh vegetables, and fruits. Eat them and listen closely. The tastes and sounds are simple and unadorned. Perhaps it's too quiet for some people who've heard nothing but the concentrated noise of sugar-fat-salt for so long. But keep listening. Soon you should hear and taste something so lovely, so easy on the ears and tongue and arteries you'll wonder how you ever lived without it.

I think of a simple serving of whole grains - boiled brown rice, barley in a soup, a bowl of oatmeal - like a solo piano piece. It can almost do everything, be an orchestra unto itself. It can establish a rhythm, create rich chords, all the while playing a melody, giving you something you recognize as a song. The British word for grain is meal, as in whole-meal bread or corn meal. Since these foods contain protein, carbohydrate, fiber, some vitamins, minerals and a little fat, whole grains come close to being whole meals.

When I eat fruits and vegetables, I hear banjos, guitars, mandolins, fiddles, and dulcimers. To me it's farm music, the romantic nostalgia about carving out a living from the land, running fingers through rich soil, working hard, sweaty brows under straw hats, reaping and sowing. It may be an anachronism given the high degree of mechanization in modern agribusiness, but I'm a pushover for those images I associate with traditional farming and the values I like to think helped build our country. Maybe I'm kidding myself, but I've done a little gardening in my time, and eating these fruits and veggies makes me feel wholesome, strong, brave, and connected to the land. I imagine a Harvest Festival hoe-down, with swinging partners around haystacks and stomping feet.

Highly refined and concentrated foods - sugar, butter, oil, salt - are so strong that they must be used judiciously. Too much and they can overpower, like the crash of the huge orchestra cymbals. A bang here and there can really help some tired, dragging pieces, but over and over again is deafening, and soon the audience can't hear anything else. Just as you can't appreciate good music above the din of too much cymbal clanging, you can't taste or benefit from good food above the noise of too-fat too-sweet.

Whole grain bread reminds me of jazz. It's full of improvisation, of musician-bakers taking a basic line and really carrying it somewhere else. You start with a simple whole grain - wheat, or rye, or barley, or oats, or rice, or millet, or all of the above - then crush, add water, yeast or sourdough, mix, knead, let rise, punch, let rise again, bake, then cool, man, cool. What you get no longer resembles what you started with, as a loaf of bread looks nothing like the kernel of wheat. It's like hearing a jazz ensemble take off on a standard tune while you sit there liking it, but puzzling until, maybe half- or three-quarters-way through a light bulb goes on and you finally recognize "April in Paris" and say, "Very tasty." Eat some just-out-of-the-oven whole grain bread, and it's the same thing: you know you like it, and are amazed that this wondrous food could come from the little kernel. Now that's cool.

Highly chemicalized, colored, and artificially preserved foods are like a completely synthesized, computer-chip-driven piece of music - the thwack and crash of the electronic percussion, the airy superficiality of the keyboard notes. It can fool some people temporarily, let them mistake the lush sounds for real violins, but eventually it's too unreal, not grounded, and not satisfying. Once in a while, I can tolerate a small dose, but not a steady diet. I know I've had too much when I start yearning to hear fingers squeaking on strings, or breath inside flutes and recorders, or actual wooden sticks on skins. It's like the yearning for real food after eating something sweetened with coal-tar-derived saccharin and colored with something red that a child relates to her crayon box.

Meats and dairy products are heavy, the bottom, the *basso profunda*. I'm talking here about tuba, double bass, maybe a little cello. These are concentrated foods, too, like the sugars and oils, since the animal was concentrating protein and fat in its flesh or with carbohydrate in its milk. Just like the sweets and fats, we only need a little taste here and there. Small doses should be enough to ground us, to anchor us after the fruity flutes and vegetable violins have been floating somewhere in the ether. But alone, or too prominent, or unbalanced by other instruments and they can sink you like the proverbial millstone. I remember as a child watching uncles go to the living room and collapse on couches and armchairs to sleep off a big Thanksgiving or Christmas dinner. Arrange wisely, here. Work in small amounts of these foods when and where needed, but not as the main part of any piece.

When I'm planning what to eat, I'm the composer and arranger, but when I cook I'm the conductor. The rhythmic sound of cleaver on wood during vegetable chopping is the percussion, and the hissing pots my wind instruments. I wave my wooden spoon, calling for crescendo, then decrescendo, pianissimo, then forte, FORTE! It all comes together and sounds like dinner. But it's not just dinner music which just accompanies a meal, it's food that becomes music. All the ingredients - whole grains, beans, fresh vegetables and fruits, and small portions of meat and dairy products - are there for you to compose, arrange, and conduct into the music that will grace your plate, satisfy your palate, and soothe the savage disease-beast you were creating from the noise of your former diet. Keep playing the new song, and make the monster go away. You know it has to come eventually, at the finale, but there's no reason to bring it on any sooner. Let the show go on the way you originally planned it. Let your new dinner music help you live your dreams.

CHAPTER 3

UNMASK THE MASQUERADER

When my children were infants and I heard one of them cry, I remember going through a mental checklist. Is the baby hurt? Perhaps her foot is caught between the crib bars or tangled in a blanket or she was hit in the face by a fallen mobile. Maybe she dropped a favorite toy or stuffed animal and can't reach it. Does she have a gas pain or some colic or simply need to be held? Perhaps her diaper needs to be changed. After addressing all of the above, if the baby was still crying, it usually meant only one thing: hungry.

My wife Kathy was an expert at knowing whether or not our babies were really hungry. She would recall when the baby last ate, and often knew it to the minute. Since she nursed both our girls, she felt a symbiotic fullness in her breasts which let her know what the cry meant (Kathy was usually crying, too, to relieve that fullness). We even thought we could identify a particular hungry cry.

An infant's hunger is a beautiful and miraculous phenomenon. When I consider how much I've had to read and study to learn what, when, and how to eat, I feel humbled and amazed by the instinct which produces the baby's plaintive howl, followed by the rooting around for and finally latching onto a nipple. With breast-feeding, it is perhaps even more wondrous because of the mystery - you never see the food. The baby simply lets go when she's had enough, but no one can see or know exactly how much she ate since there aren't any hash marks or measurement lines on a breast.

A baby's hunger is urgent. The metabolic fires are raging so she can double her birth weight in six months and triple it in a year. That's a lot of work, and it requires a lot of energy and building blocks. No wonder she cries that way when she's hungry. We must remember, though, that this period of intense energy-need and rapid growth ends pretty quickly. People can't keep tripling their weight every year, although some go on eating as if the growth curve never flattens out, and they continue to grow horizontally.

I remember watching each of my children breast-feed and thinking, "Enjoy it, honey, it will never be easier." They seemed to know exactly what they needed, how much, and how often. I envied this, because I was more often clue-less about quantity and frequency. I was often aware of eating because it was time to do it or because, like Mount Everest, it was there. As for quantity, I'd often finish whatever was on the plate no matter how loaded it was, and sometimes found myself going faster so I wouldn't get full before the plate was cleaned. Sometimes I had the insight that what I experienced as hunger was a masquerader wearing a hunger-mask. It might have been some other problem I unconsciously converted into hunger, such as anxiety, depression, low self-esteem, anger, boredom, frustration, job dissatisfaction, marital discord, unemployment, grief, or disappointment. These are often difficult or require a lot of work to fix. But if my subconscious masks these problems by turning them into hunger, I might mistakenly believe that eating is the way to feel better. This is not only easier, but even temporarily effective, since a full belly almost always soothes me. The unresolved stressor remains, though, and in my imagination I hear it laugh and say, "The disguise worked."

The feel-good is an illusion and only adds to the problem, layering an eating disorder with all its potential health complications onto the primary mood disorder or the lost job or the interpersonal conflict. When I gained weight and my clothes got tight, it made my mood even worse, and I see this frequently in my patients, too. Sherry admits, "I eat when I'm depressed," then gets more depressed when she steps on the scale. Leonard eats when he's anxious, especially about his work, and he can polish off a large bag of corn chips while driving to a sales call he's worried about. I find him overweight with mildly elevated blood pressure and counsel him to watch the snack foods, but he says he gets "really hungry" while he's working, and believes that the mental energy he expends increases his need for calories. I try to orient him to the reality that his weight gain means he is eating beyond his imagined needs.

Dysfunctional is a common word in pop-psychology, but it's a good term for the response to false hunger. To help fix things and get us back to our diet homes, we need to be able to recognize real hunger, to distinguish it from the pain that often wears a hunger costume. We have to learn how to unmask the masquerader, to hear our own crying and know which one is the real hungry cry. Whenever I feel the urge to eat something, I try to ask three questions which resemble my old mental checklist when the babies cried. What came before the hunger? What comes with the hunger? What comes after the hunger?

I've found that real hunger is more likely to be preceded by a period of fasting. If I wake up ravenous and it's been twelve or fourteen hours since my last meal, it's probably the real thing, and breakfast is truly breaking the fast. But if the hunger alarms sounds only a short time after a meal or snack, such as within an hour or two, it may be a masquerader. I imagine Kathy hearing the baby cry and saying, "She can't be hungry, I just fed her," then say that to myself. This rule doesn't always hold, though. I have some patients who eat very low fat diets or have esophageal reflux (a condition in which stomach acid flows backwards and burns the esophagus) who may need to eat small meals frequently, such as five or six times a day. This is especially true if they couple a low fat diet with a huge calorie-deficit from vigorous activity, such as the man I cared for who rode his bicycle to work every day, a thirty-mile round trip. He was very lean and needed to nibble all day long, which he called "grazing".

Perhaps it's most important to look at what comes with the hunger and ask what other feelings or emotions or hurts might be behind the mask. Is there anxiety or boredom? Does eating fill some momentary void or emptiness? Does it postpone or delay some unpleasant task or project? Now I can readily identify the nervous eaters in my practice since I've been there. I used to make characteristic pantry-raids whenever I had writer's block, hoping the food would transmute into words. I would stand at the kitchen counter holding a bag or box of something, stare into space, and mechanically shovel in my snack. But I discovered later that I didn't need to eat to relieve the obstruction, only to get away from the task and do something else for a time. A brisk walk, a few push-ups, pushing the vacuum cleaner a half-hour or so, or a couple of mindless minutes in front of the tube work as well for me.

Finally, we should examine our feelings after hunger and eating, looking for satisfaction or a persistent vague sense of an unfulfilled need. If I have the urge to eat again within thirty minutes or so, I probably wasn't hungry in the first place but was fooled by the masquerader. I usually feel embarrassed after this happens, but if I can recall that feeling the next time I may be able to stop myself before I eat something I don't need.

I've also found that real hunger is much harder to distract than an imitator. Consider the hungry crying infant again. You can shake toys in her face and rock her and change her and swing her and stroll her, but only food will put out the fire. False hunger is usually easier to handle by taking a walk or bike ride, reading a book, paying some bills, or making a telephone call. If you can't distract it and the timing is right then you may actually be hungry. Go ahead, then. Eat. Enjoy. But remember, real hunger is usually easy to satisfy with reasonable amounts of food. If you gorge and stuff yourself it may mean that something other than hunger has contaminated the real thing.

A twelve- or fourteen-hour overnight fast can be good training to better recognize real hunger. It has helped me to get to know how it feels and what it means when the stomach growls voraciously and says, "Break-fast, break-fast." Every other hunger pang should feel the same, like a fire in the belly, started by the part of the brain that knows you need fuel or building blocks. It's a primitive drive that, if need be, can move you blindly, single-mindedly, and passionately in search of food as it does for the hungry infant. It's a gift.

Get to know that little baby inside you. When you hear crying, go through the list. See if your emotional foot is stuck between the crib bars of a trapped life. Try to solve your problems, but if you can't do so quickly or easily, don't delude yourself into thinking that the transient pleasure you derive from eating will do anything but give you more problems.

If the false urge resists and won't go away, fight it. Wrestle it to the ground, pull off the mask and say, "So it was you, Boredom. I wasn't hungry at all." Then give it the old Frederick March to Humphrey Bogart line from the end of *The Desperate Hours*: "Get out of my house."

Everyone has heard "Don't live to eat, eat to live." When you've ruled out all the pretenders and are truly hungry, recognize it and be grateful for the wondrous gift of appetite. Eat heartily. Savor every mouthful. But when you're done, be done, and get on with the rest of your life.

CHAPTER 4

BLIZZARD OF '79

I've had a particular affection for Kathy's split pea soup ever since I found it at the end of a long snow-covered road.

It was February, 1979 and snowing hard. I was an intern standing in our lounge at about 4:00 p.m. saying goodbye to my friend and fellow-intern, Ted, who told me I had a thing for snow. He recalled a similar farewell during a blizzard the previous winter when we were fourth-year medical students and he was preparing to go home before the roads became impassable, while I stayed behind, assigned to "cover the house" - spend the night in the hospital and respond to whatever emergencies arose. "Here we go again," he said, except that this time I only needed to stay until 7:00 p.m. when Gary, our classmate, relieved me. Ted predicted that Gary wouldn't show because the old car which had carried him the many miles through college and medical school could go any time. He said that a major snowstorm like the one we were having would be the stress to throw off the car's delicate equilibrium, strand Gary somewhere on the road, and strand me in the hospital. I had worked plenty of twenty-four and thirty-six hour shifts before, but when it's snowing as hard as it was that day and you're tired and hungry with a new wife waiting in your apartment, there is a sense of urgency to get out and get home.

At five o'clock I stood in the telephone operators' booth and looked out the huge window that overlooked the doctors' parking lot, watching the snow pile up. I took an informal unscientific poll among a few nurses, the Emergency Room orderly, and a security guard asking, "Do you think he'll show?" They all said "yes", but no one sounded too convincing. At five-thirty the operator suggested I call and let him know I was anxious to get going, and ask him to get in earlier if possible. I decided not to, saying, "He'll be here."

At six forty-five I had just finished examining someone in the Intensive Care Unit, and everything was fairly quiet in the hospital. Ignoring the possible jinx I was creating, I started loading up my backpack and getting ready to go. At six fifty-nine I walked back to the operators' booth to watch and wait. It was dark outside, but huge floodlights shone on the lot and illuminated the rather vigorous snowfall. I had on hats, boots, gloves, and coat and had written a detailed note for Gary explaining which patients might need special attention over the next few hours. At seven o'clock exactly, his old car rattled effortlessly into the parking lot on tire chains. "You made it," I said and thanked him profusely. "Did you ever doubt me?" he asked. "Not for a minute," I told him.

I called Kathy to tell her I was on my way. She wondered if the trolleys would still be running, because the news was reporting that a lot of public transportation had already been shut down. "They'll be running," I said, feeling that if I had been lucky enough to leave, I'd make it home with no problem, too. I started walking the hundred or so yards to the trolley stop, all downhill and a little precarious, so I moved slowly. The snow was deeper than I had anticipated which slowed me even more. Then I heard a rumbling. Thunder, I hoped, or wind, or maybe a distant snowplow, but no such luck. It was the trolley, speeding through the stop where I was not yet waiting, just fifty yards away. I finally got there and stared at the tracks in disbelief. The prudent option would have been to turn around and walk back to the hospital and spend the night there. "No way," I thought, "I'm going home," and started walking along the tracks in case another trolley came along.

It took me fifteen minutes to walk to the next stop at the shopping mall. It was eerily quiet, except for the snowplows working the parking lot. I accepted the reality that no more trolleys would come along for a while, if ever, so I walked out to the highway to continue my journey on foot with another three miles till home.

The snow was above my knees and I fell twice in huge drifts. The second time I lay there laughing a few minutes, feeling ridiculous. After walking another half mile or so, I heard another rumbling from something small coming down the road without flashing lights, so it wasn't a plow or emergency vehicle. Incredibly enough it was a car, and I wondered what kind of nut was out driving on such a night. Then I recalled that I had hitched a ride in the blizzard the year before, and remembered telling my friends the following day that a unique camaraderie develops instantly between people who meet under those circumstances. I stuck out a stubby gloved thumb, and the car stopped, of course. Inside was a perfectly normal-looking middle-aged man, driving an old Ford with no snow tires and no chains and built before front-wheel and four-wheel drive were as common as today.

He had driven out to the building supply store where they were supposed to be having a sale but, "Do you believe it," he said, "they were closed," surprised that since he was out, why weren't they. He dropped me off about a mile from home, and I found myself energized and walking faster and faster as I got closer. I finally stepped into the apartment, covered head to toe in snow. My beard was one huge ice crystal from frozen condensed out-breaths. "My abominable snowman," Kathy said as we embraced. I pulled back from the hug and lifted my nose. "What's that smell?" I asked. "Is it what I think it is?" I walked dripping into the kitchen and lifted the pot lid to find my reward for trudging home. It was a hearty pot of soup, made with green split peas, onions, carrots, and celery, in a stock from the water we saved from steaming vegetables. She'd also made some short-grain brown rice, steamed kale dressed with apple cider vinegar and dill, and croutons for the soup made from toasted cubes of whole-wheat sourdough bread.

At that moment it was the most wholesome and satisfying meal I had ever eaten. I had three helpings of everything, then sank into the sofa with a full belly and a good physical tired in my legs, and started describing my journey home as waves of sweet sleep rolled over me.

$$\boxed{\text{CHAPTER 5}}$$

NO RULES, ONLY TWEAKS

I've eliminated all diet-rules from my way of eating. I no longer think in terms of can and can't or should and shouldn't. My only relevant question is whether or not something is truly a food and not some completely chemicalized laboratory creation. All real food becomes fair game, and then the only critical issues are quantity (how much) and frequency (how often).

I used to think of some foods as poisons and imagined skulls and crossbones on items such as ice cream, french fries, red meat, cakes, cookies, and anything refined or processed. My diet became progressively narrow, which my body liked as it slimmed down and my blood lost cholesterol and I got fewer respiratory infections. But the rest of my life became narrower, too, as I found myself avoiding activities where I couldn't eat the way I wanted. Emotionally I didn't appreciate what my body was enjoying so much. I had painted myself into a very tiny corner, only agreeing to go certain places or see certain people, because so many social functions involved food.

At one point in the early 1980's I was following a very strict Macrobiotic diet which advised against eating any tropical fruits because they don't grow in the temperate climate where I lived. It didn't make any scientific sense since oranges and bananas contained vitamin C and potassium, but Macrobiotics was more philosophically-based, and maintained that some immeasurable balance was disturbed when we ate foods that didn't or couldn't grow in our climatic region. I remember attending a party given by someone who adhered to this same principle where someone said, "It's so nice to be able to go out and be served a fruit salad and not have to worry about picking out the oranges." I agreed and so did some others. As I think about it now, though, I see myself as arrogant, self-righteous, and ridiculous since I was judging other people and often thinking less of them because they ate eggs, steak, chocolate cookies, cheese, and oranges, but never ate brown rice. I had reduced all the beauty and wonder of humanity to a simplistic evaluation of what people put in their mouths, and thereby deprived myself of a whole lot more than a few extra calories.

Years later, as part of my formal Preventive Medicine training, I discovered some real poisons when I studied Toxicology and learned about substances such as mercury, lead, arsenic, PCB's, dioxin, and botulinum toxin (the substance produced by the bacteria which causes botulism). One of the core concepts in Toxicology is that everything is a poison and potentially toxic depending on the dose. At some low dose, almost every poison is safe, and at some high dose, almost every safe substance is poison. Even familiar friends can cause problems in specific instances, as when a patient with congestive heart failure is water-intoxicated, or a person with emphysema is made worse when too much oxygen suppresses the drive to breathe.

At the same time I took a critical look at my own behavior, as I smugly and easily avoided all the bad stuff - red meat, dairy products, sugar - and, because I had formerly been quite a glutton, enjoyed the way people marveled at my new-found self-control. Self-control? Hardly. I had simply transferred my piggishness to the good stuff, gorging myself on whole grains, veggies and so-called natural cookies and cakes (made with whole wheat flour instead of bleached white, oil instead of butter, and honey or barley malt instead of white sugar). I was still a pig, just with safer food.

When I finally decided it was time to stop being a pig I came up with No Rules, Only Tweaks. Nothing is good or bad, and I don't go on and off any foods, but simply tweak my diet depending on the situation. Most days I tweak fairly narrow, keeping my diet centered around whole grains, beans, fresh vegetables and fruits. Other times I tweak it rather wide, as when I'm a guest in someone's home and enjoy small servings of chicken and even a buttery sugary dessert. I stopped being afraid of certain foods. I began to relate to meat, fat, and sugar with less fear and more respect for their flavor and power. I respect them so much that I don't eat them very often, and when I do it's very small amounts, as when I have a tiny sliver of God-knows-what's-in-it birthday cake at a person's home, or a nibble or two of chicken at a restaurant. When the cake is whole-grain-fruit-juice-sweetened-fat-free, I can polish off two or three mammoth hunks. When the entree is brown rice stir fry, I can put away the whole pot. I don't mind holding onto a little fear for the old regulars, since I've found it a good way to finally control my tendency to overeat.

Don't let me mislead you. My diet is still very limited compared to what I see friends, family, co-workers, and patients eat, but I do enjoy little tastes here and there of some things I would have never touched just a few years ago. There's no rule anymore that says I can't, and that makes a huge difference. I see it as deciding who's in charge, as the difference between being free or in diet-prison where you're forbidden to eat certain foods, where the diet is as rigid as jail bars, or as black and white as convict stripes. A free person can eat whatever he or she wants, as long as the quantity and frequency are appropriate. A free person is flexible and sees more color. I needed this change in orientation because there is always some party, business dinner, or wedding reception when I am confronted with having to or wanting to eat something with relatively high toxicity which I have come to believe is bad for me.

About fifteen years ago some good friends invited Kathy and me to dinner and served a spinach soufflé that was loaded with eggs and cheese. The cook announced that she had made it especially for me since I was a vegetarian. I could have explained that there were different types of vegetarians, and that in fact I wasn't a vegetarian since I ate fish once or twice a month, but never touched dairy products or eggs. To prevent a major embarrassment and insure that Kathy would continue to speak to me, I ate and enjoyed a small serving. This reinforced my freedom, because I had made a case-specific decision and wasn't following some hard and fast rule. Since I had kept the dose low it didn't hurt me in any obvious way - I didn't have a runny nose the next day, and if my cholesterol level jumped overnight, it was back into the low-to-mid-hundreds the next time I checked it. This reinforced the notion that something I had formerly considered poison could be completely benign if I knew how to use it.

No Rules, Only Tweaks means that as long as you know how much and how often, you can eat anything. The only catch is that you'll have to learn from experience as I have. I can point you in the right direction, out of the woods, but can't and won't give you the specific hard numbers, ounces, milligrams, percentages, or tell you exactly what to do. Tweaking is a very personal thing. But if you're anything like the people I talk to every day in my office, you already know what to do with a left brain full of facts and figures about fats, fiber, and fish oil. You should also have an awareness of personal needs, risks, and desired outcomes such as weight, waist size, blood pressure, cholesterol level, family history, energy level, skin condition, and other health concerns. All you need now is the how, a way to get at all that stored information when you need it and let it direct your behavior when the spirit is sleeping and the flesh is weak. The right brain diet directions in this book will be your key to unlock the door on the left, so that both sides of the brain together can guide you safely all the way home. The dietary winds may blow hard at times trying to break you, but if you know how to tweak you'll bend instead.

CHAPTER 6

SWEAT FOOD

The word convenient comes from two Latin roots that mean *come together*, and our current use suggests something that comes together fairly easily. Trains and planes and automobiles make it convenient for us to move from place to place, reducing what formerly took days or weeks or months and turning it into hours. Telephones, FAX machines, and computers make communication more convenient, and the evolving information superhighway makes it even easier in some ways. Modern energy production makes it more convenient for most people to light, heat, cool, clean, and cook in their living spaces. Even home entertainment can be as quick and easy as a telephone call for a cable movie order.

We also have convenience foods, often sold in convenience stores, which make it easier for us to get what is usually advertised as nourishing. When I talk to people who live harried, hurried lives they usually consider these a blessing. Todd and Barbara are a couple I've seen in my office who are thirty-eight, both work, and have two children ages seven and nine. They tell me they couldn't survive without frozen entrees, their microwave, and fast food. They try to make better choices more often - light and lean meals and salads - but admit that they still feel forced at times to sacrifice quality for speed and peace when their kids whine for the burgers, fries, and milkshakes they've seen on TV. Todd also tells me that when he's at the counter paying for that quick morning eye-opening cup of coffee, it's just too easy to pick up a high fat high sugar sweet roll at the same time. His use of "quick" for the coffee and "just too easy to pick up" are key, because he'll tell me in the next breath that he knows he "shouldn't indulge." I think he's trying to tell me that if it wasn't so easy, he wouldn't do it, that the convenience somehow takes away his ability to choose.

We used to be separated from today's convenience foods by natural barriers of labor and access, because it was harder to get and/or harder to make the high fat high sugar items that have the most potential to harm us. Let's say, it's two hundred years ago and you want some cake. What do you do? You would probably have to make it yourself, and it might involve grinding the wheat, milking the cow, churning the butter, and splitting the wood to fire up the oven. These are all barriers of labor, intrinsic obstacles of work which keep you from immediately gratifying your desire for something sweet and rich. Even if you didn't have to grow it or milk it or churn it yourself, you'd probably have to travel by horse or coach or wagon to the nearest town for supplies, or to find a bakery, which will also keep you from getting the quick sugar-fix exactly when you want it. I consider my eating behavior sophisticated, but even I occasionally yield to convenience. Like Todd, when I'm at the natural foods store counter paying for my lentils and organic carrots, it's just too easy to pick up a carob chip crisp brown rice treat or a jumbo fat-free but calorie-rich oatmeal cookie. I looked for a way to minimize the negative effects of convenience and decided to re-construct some barriers of labors and access. I wanted to spend more time and do more work to get foods with concentrated fat and sugar, and hoped that this would allow me more space to reflect on what I was doing.

One of the first foods I addressed was peanut butter, something I had always loved and was practically weaned on like a lot of other baby-boomers. But peanut butter is high in fat, even though it's vegetable fat with a relatively high proportion of safe mono-unsaturates. Commercial brands had added fat and sugar, and natural food store brands were expensive. There were also warnings about possible contamination with aflatoxin, a carcinogen produced by a mold often found on peanuts. For all these reasons, I decided to make my own and only eat what I produced myself. It would be fresher, I could inspect every peanut to make sure none was moldy, and I could feel good about this homey activity, making something from scratch in my own kitchen. The only thing I wasn't doing was growing the peanuts.

I learned that even with a high-power food processor, it's a lot of work to make peanut butter if you're shelling the nuts and taking the time to look at each one. Ever try to fill just one cup with shelled peanuts when you're cracking them yourself? It takes a while. Then how much peanut butter do you think you get for that cup of nuts? I got half a cup, but it was precious to me. I rationed it because I didn't want to go through the trouble of making it again any time soon. I had learned how to spread peanut butter from television commercials where brown creamy tidal waves roll over sliced white bread. Of course, the manufacturers want us to use tons of the stuff, then run back to the market for more. In my kitchen, the tidal wave looked more like a puddle.

I had separated myself from overeating a delicious but high-fat food with a self-imposed barrier of labor. I didn't tell myself I wasn't allowed to eat it since I could have as much as I wanted, as long as I made it. I just didn't feel like making it very often, so I chose to eat less.

I learned a similar lesson about maple syrup. I love maple syrup which, like peanut butter, is a uniquely American food, a New World discovery. Whenever I eat pancakes with maple syrup, I conjure up images of George Washington's soldiers wintering at Valley Forge making fire cakes, pouring crude batter onto hot rocks, then topping it off with a liquid confection they had learned to make from the local natives. Pure maple syrup is expensive, but there's nothing else like it.

I attended an outdoor seminar on maple syruping in late winter, 1979, at a local arboretum. The arboretum director taught us shivering students how to identify sugar maple trees by their small

February buds, how to tap the trees, collect the sap, and boil it down into syrup. The instructor recommended boiling it outside, since the process generates huge amounts of steam which can ruin kitchen walls. They told us it takes about forty gallons of sap to make one gallon of syrup. I was fascinated enough to buy a few taps in the arboretum store and waited until late February when conditions in southeastern Pennsylvania are likely to be ideal - below-freezing nights when the sap collects in the lowest parts of the tree, and above-freezing days when the sap rises to feed the tender young buds which have to become leaves and seeds. That's when you drive in the tap and collect (short-circuit) the sap.

I still had one major hurdle - no maple trees - since I was a newly married intern living in an apartment. Kathy's parents, however, lived nearby, and had a few maples large enough to tap. My parents were also close, and they had an outdoor brick fireplace/barbecue area. So there it was - a sap source and a work station. The only thing left was to find the time, since timing and temperature are everything in maple sugaring. When the sap rises, you have to be ready. Most interns don't have much time but, luckily, I was in the middle of a four-week stint of night-shifts at the hospital where I'd work from 7:00 p.m. to 7:00 a.m., then be off the next day until 7:00 p.m. It worked out perfectly. I'd finish work in the morning, go collect sap in large plastic jugs from my in-laws' trees, then drive to my parents' place. There, puffy-eyed and sleep-deprived, over an outdoor wood fire, in a huge spaghetti pot, I boiled down about four gallons of watery, tasteless sap into approximately a cup and a half of sweet, thick, smoke-flavored, holy maple syrup. I had it for months, using only precious drops at a time.

Does this mean that everyone has to make their own cakes or peanut butter or maple syrup? No, of course not. But it certainly wouldn't hurt to make more things from scratch. The real point is to eat *as if* you had to make it yourself, knowing you would have to make more when you ran out. Also, it takes labor and energy to make food, which I found out when I made my peanut butter and maple syrup. We need to respect that labor and energy and recognize that some foods require more than others. Farming is hard work, even by modern, mechanized means, but that may be just the beginning. If the food goes directly to market, then the only extra energy is whatever it takes to box and ship it and put it in the shelves. But if it goes to a factory to be cooked, canned, frozen, or refined, the extra human and machine labor makes the energy costs rise dramatically.

I've observed that the foods with the most potential to harm us are usually the ones that have been processed the most, by such methods as extracting, refining, concentrating, all of which require energy and increase caloric density. Maple syrup is an extracted, refined, concentrated part of maple sap. The sap is like water, while the syrup is thick and sugar-rich. I worked hard for the batch I produced in 1979, and nowadays I try to remember how much work (and fun) it was so that I'll respect that, and only use it sparingly. Similarly, table and baking sugar are extracted, refined, concentrated parts of sugar cane or sugar beets, and it took energy to make them. Any oil is an extracted, concentrated, refined part of seeds, grains, nuts, or fruits, and butter is an extracted, concentrated, refined part of whole milk.

Today we use machinery and electrical energy from fossil fuels or nuclear reactions to do the work, but hundreds of years ago it was human hands and energy. When we use human energy to make food, we burn the calories before we've even eaten and create a deficit we can safely and deliciously satisfy at the table. Only a tablespoon of butter or oil contains a whopping one hundred or more calories. If we pre-burn those calories churning or pounding seeds, we come out even. But when we let the manufacturer's machines and fossil fuels do our work for us, the energy we consume ends up on our abdomens, thighs, and buttocks, stored there and waiting for the burn that never comes.

So re-build a few barriers. Make more things from scratch. Find a store you can walk to when you want a snack, and imagine yourself going into the fields to gather food. Imagine yourself cracking and grinding nuts with large stones the next time you want to eat something with a lot of oil, then eat a little less. Think of me on a cold February morning, wood smoke irritating my red up-all-night eyes the next time you pour the maple syrup, and pour a little less.

Eat food that contains your sweat, effort, imagination, and creativity. Let food become your consuming art, not just an object to consume. Let's eat as if life was a little less convenient, food was a little less abundant, and life and food were a little more precious. Maybe it will make life last a little longer.

CHAPTER 7

SCHEMATIC AND TRANSFORMED PLANTS

Dietary advice has come in different shapes and forms the past forty years. In 1956, the U.S. Department of Agriculture gave it to us on paper, advising Americans to eat something from each of these four food groups every day - meats, dairy products, vegetables and fruits, and breads and cereals. These groups became known as the Basic Four and held up until 1977 when a U.S. Senate sub-committee chaired by George McGovern published *Dietary Goals for the United States.* This report along with Surgeon General Julius Richmond's *Healthy People* in 1979 suggested that the overconsumption of high-fat meats and milk-derived foods could increase the risk of developing heart disease, the nation's number one killer, as well as cancers such as colon, uterus, and possibly breast and prostate.

I appreciated these reports which hit the Government Printing Office bookshelves at the same time I was finishing my training and starting in practice, but didn't notice much impact on the patients I was seeing. I frequently asked them what they ate or had them keep diet diaries, especially interested in how they planned their main daily meal, what they thought represented balance. Typically I saw or heard people choose some type of meat first - beef or chicken mostly, occasionally fish or pork - often referring to it as "the protein". Next they'd talk about a starch, either potatoes in some form (baked, mashed, roasted, fried),or noodles or rice. Finally they'd include a green vegetable, and the ones I heard about most often were iceberg lettuce, spinach, and string beans. This was the predominate model, with the occasional cabbage and Brussels sprout enthusiasts.

Many of my patients respond differently in 1997 when I ask the same questions. They're more likely to specify skinless chicken rather than red meat, their potatoes are usually baked instead of fried, and often dressed with a non-fat sour cream. The iceberg lettuce is still around, but I see more people getting into romaine and other darker greens and using low-fat, fat-free, or at worst an olive oil-based salad dressing. I attribute these changes to ongoing Public Health education by groups such as the American Heart Association, the National Cholesterol Education program, and again the Department of Agriculture which figuratively carved its advice in stone by giving us the food pyramid in 1992. While the Basic Four safely hedged by telling us to eat a little of everything, the pyramid graphically advises that we prioritize our diet choices according to their relative importance or ability to harm. Grains, breads, and cereals form the solid foundation, with vegetables and fruits at the next level. Meats, sweets, and oils are at or near the narrower apex, indicating that we can eat them, but in smaller amounts than the foods at the base.

I've seen the pyramid in and on everything from medical textbooks to cereal boxes. I like the visual impact, the immediate message to eat more of what's at the bottom and less of what's at the top. But I don't like the metaphor, the notion that dietary advice is entombed with mummified bodies and old bones. I'd prefer something a little more lively. It's also still a little too left-brained for me, spelling out what to eat by food categories and numbers of daily servings, so I asked my right brain for some other image to cue proper eating. It gave me the schematic plant - a collection of foods which together figuratively resemble an entire plant. It has roots, stalks, stems, leaves, flowers, fruits, and seeds. I'm sure this is a gross oversimplification, but my right brain license lets me take liberties with formal botany. I try to eat something from every part of the plant every day, which automatically covers the most important bottom pyramid sections. They don't all need to be present at the same meal (although my day's main meal usually contains each one), but I think of a daily plate, the combination of everything I eat in one day as having to contain all parts of a plant.

Each part of my schematic plant has a different job. Roots dive deep into rich soil with little hairy arms that snake into dark places looking for water and minerals. Leaves are often broad and flat, unfolding and spreading out in the sunshine to soak up the radiant energy and change it into food. Stalks and stems transport what the roots and leaves picked up and manufactured. The fruits and flowers package the payload - the seeds. They have to have (singly or in combination) sweetness, fragrance, or beauty to attract seed-spreading critters - bugs or birds or beasts - so the plant can re-establish itself. Nasturtiums and day lilies are edible flowers, but we also eat flower buds as broccoli (those little green buds on the head open into yellow flowers if the stalk isn't harvested).

Seeds are the small, compact, concentrated packets that carry the energy and information necessary to make a new plant. I think of them as the most important parts of my schematic plant, because without them, the plant can't reproduce. They are usually very durable, with a protective coat, and able to survive long periods if conditions are right (some seeds recovered from Egyptian tombs sprouted after thousands of years of storage).

The roots I eat most often are carrots, which I consider a staple. Occasionally I'll substitute or add turnips, radishes, or parsnips. Thanks to my Macrobiotic education I discovered another root vegetable called burdock. It has an unusual but satisfying earthy flavor (my friend Jim says it tastes like dirt) and grows wild in much of eastern North America along roadsides and at the edge of wooded areas. I've dug up my share on foraging forays and so understand why Macrobiotic teacher Michio Kushi says that burdock makes you strong twice – once when you dig, and once when you eat. It's easier to find now in natural foods markets. Tubers (potatoes) and bulbs (onions) aren't really roots even though they grow underground. I think of them as free foods, to be included if I want, but most times not to substitute for any other schematic category. This is why I'll frequently have potatoes and grains at the same meal. They both provide complex carbohydrate as starch, but represent different plant parts.

Like the patients from my early years in practice, I grew up thinking that green vegetables meant iceberg lettuce, spinach, or peas. Now when I think of greens I look for a dark green lettuce such as romaine, or preferably something hardier I have to cook such as kale, collards or cabbage. Spinach and its relative swiss chard are good choices too, although I avoid them because their high oxalic acid content increases my risk to manufacture more kidney stones (one was enough for me). I don't think of stalks and stems as major categories, and find it easier to eat them as part of leaves since they usually come attached. When I have them separately, such as celery or asparagus, I once again see them as free choices, but not substitutes for other greens.

Fruits are familiar enough, but the list should include squashes and pumpkins which are actually the fruits of flowering vines and related to melons, even though I usually think of them as vegetables. Tomatoes, peppers, and eggplants are fruits, too, although some people avoid these and potatoes because they are in the so-called nightshade family - botanical cousins of the poisonous plant belladonna - and were linked to joint complaints twenty years ago by horticulturist Norman Childers.

Seeds include whole grains and beans. Grains, the seeds of cereal grasses, have been human staples for ten thousand years and include rice, wheat, barley, oats, rye, millet, corn, amaranth, sorghum, and others - different ones in different locales. Beans are the dried seeds of leguminous plants, and they, too, have been part of human diets for centuries, often complementing the grains in such cuisine as Native American (corn and pinto beans), Middle Eastern (chickpeas and bulgur wheat), Oriental (rice and soybeans).

Every grain has three parts. The bran is the durable, outer, skin-like coat which provides the fiber. The germ is the seed of the seed, the part that will sprout to make a new plant and contains protein, essential fats, and vitamin E. The endosperm or starchy part is the stored food for the new plant and provides the carbohydrates or energy. In whole grains, all three parts are present. Refined grains usually just have the starchy part, such as white rice, white bread, white pasta, degerminated cornmeal, and most cold cereals. The other two parts should not be excluded. Patients have described their attempts to achieve dietary balance by sprinkling bran and germ into meatloaf and casseroles. This is one way to do it suppose, but I'd rather eat the whole grains themselves since everything's already there.

The patients I counsel can be anything from strict vegans (eating only plant-derived foods) to those who will eat just about anything but try to include more whole grains, vegetables, and fruits to complement their meat and dairy products. In between are those who tend to be mostly vegetarian, but occasionally eat fish and/or chicken and/or low fat dairy foods. Anyone who avoids all animal-derived foods should ensure adequate Vitamin B12 intake, either from fermented soybean products such as miso or tempeh, or through supplementation (a consultation with a nutritionist may be helpful here).

I occasionally eat some fish or poultry, but still think of them as plants, only transformed. Most animal tissue was ultimately derived from plants the animal ate directly or indirectly, as when a carnivore lion eats a herbivore gazelle. No matter what you eat, there's a plant somewhere down the food chain. While I eat a schematic plant every day, I eat transformed plants anywhere from two to three times a week to two to three times a month. It tends to be more when I dine out or over holidays, but I frequently go several weeks without any. On the days I eat some meat, I make beans optional since I don't need them for the protein.

So without looking at books or pyramids, I think of my schematic plant and check a mental list every day. Did I eat whole grains at every meal, with complementary beans at least once? What fruits and flowers did I eat, and what roots and leaves? Usually I can fill in the blank for every one of these questions, although the plant I create may look a little unusual. Sometimes it's a carrot with collard greens coming out the top and a long vine extending up holding a butternut squash, inside of which is lentils and brown rice as seeds. I think of it as an artistic statement, a surrealist's approach to eating. Sometimes a bizarre, transformed, almost unrecognizable plant with fins or feathers swims or steps onto the canvas.

When I eat the whole plant, I feel like I become every part: dark, strong, deep and mysterious as roots; broad and wide as leaves, able to unfold when I need to soak up heat or light; sweet, pretty, fragrant, and attractive as flowers and fruits; compact, smart, durable, and energetic as seeds. When I eat a whole plant, I become a whole person.

CHAPTER 8

VACATION AND HOMECOMING - 1980

Kathy and I decided to make the trip and get it out of our systems before we had children. Our friends Jim and Carol agreed and we all drove off into the wilds of central Maine for a summer vacation. It was a cabin on an island on a lake with no plumbing or electricity, and a pit privy about ten yards away - outside, in the woods. We packed the car with supplies - grains and beans mostly, since we planned to get some vegetables and fruits along the way. We also brought two cases of beer, which I called the liquid grains.

We had looked forward to getting away from the craziness of the megalopolis, living clean, eating clean, swimming, hiking, reading, writing, and coming home refreshed and renewed. After three days, we were tired of brown rice and oatmeal and split peas and kidney beans, had drunk all the beer, and found it impossible to hike without toxic doses of insect repellent. We packed up and headed for the seashore resorts of southeast Maine, looking for the civilized, pampered life in a hotel or motel where we could get a shower (first one in four days unless you count the dip in the lake), then have a relaxing meal somewhere prepared by someone else that didn't contain rice or beans.

The weather didn't cooperate, delivering one of those biting, cold-goes-right-through-you rains they can get in Maine in August to remind you that summer comes late to this region and leaves early.

We could barely see the hotels through the fogged windows. Every place we tried was full. We were cold, hungry, tired, and cranky (we wanted to do this before we had children, but we were playing the child-parts pretty well ourselves).

Finally we found an old hotel with lots of character and a great view of the classic rocky coastline. The registration clerk told us there were no rooms available in the main building, but she could put us up in a detached cabin they used to use as maids' quarters. There was one problem, though, she said: the rooms didn't have bathrooms. We asked if they were outside, in the woods, but she said, "No, just down the hall." "Close enough," we said, "we'll take them."

By that time we felt more hungry than dirty or tired, so we skipped the showers we'd been dreaming about and headed for food. There was one collective thought on our four famished minds – Lobster. Jim and I went back to the front desk to ask about restaurants, and the clerk recommended several popular establishments. Then Jim asked where the locals went when they wanted good, inexpensive, home-cooked meals. She directed us to a small, casual place off the main road. "It's not fancy," she told us, "but they have very good lobster."

We were not dressed or shaved or clean or patient enough for fancy or atmosphere, so we had no problem with the small brightly lit restaurant that had booths, wooden tables, and plastic tablecloths. Our orders were simple. Since we were all bone-chilled we asked for New England clam chowder, followed by lobster. I ordered tails, since I don't have the skill, patience, or desire to deal with the whole animal. The soups were hot and wonderful, made with milk and/or cream with a dollop of butter on top - all items I usually avoid, but I didn't care. Our waitress brought a basket of bread and told us they were oatmeal rolls. The name didn't fit, since oatmeal conjures up something thick and heavy, while these rolls were light enough to float away. We did find some oatmeal inside as scattered, infrequent flecks of brown, swimming in a sea of bleached white flour, yeast, and dough conditioners. Oatmeal got top billing for what was barely a cameo appearance, but we were hungry, and the bread went down easily.

As for our main courses, well, what can I say. We were in Maine, next to the ocean, eating lobster, God was in Heaven, and all was right with the world. After we were all stuffed and satisfied and swore we wouldn't eat again for days, I asked about dessert. Kathy, Jim, and Carol were surprised, since I'm usually the one who passes when everyone else goes for a taste of something sweet. I ordered a huge piece of blueberry pie, made with those small New England, short-growing-season berries, certainly containing refined white sugar, and I could taste shortening in the crust. I ate every bit and even pressed my fork onto the plate to get the crumbs. If only for the hunger, cold, fatigue, distance from home and anticipation, it was easily one of the most memorable meals we ever had (we still talk about it). We went back to the hotel and collapsed into the beds of old maids, dreaming of a tomorrow shower in a bathroom down the hall.

When we finally got home two days later we were tired of driving, being away from home, sleeping in strange beds, and eating in restaurants. We had driven six hours without stopping to eat so we were hungry, but yearned for something simple without fat, sugar, or salt. It had to be something simple, since we had cleaned out the cupboards and refrigerator before we had gone away, and even if any stores had been open that late on a Sunday night, neither of us felt like traveling even one more minute in a car.

Kathy put on a pot of short grain brown rice, the stuff we'd thought we'd had enough of several days before, but now couldn't wait to eat. We had to have some, since we consider it the simplest, most wonderful, healing food we know, and the best thing to travel East to West since Marco Polo brought back noodles. I scrounged up an onion, a couple of softening carrots, and a browning hunk of savoy cabbage. They would have to do, but they did quite nicely. After boiling the veggies, I added a little miso (fermented soy paste) to the water to make broth, which we drank first and felt instantly purified. Next we ate the rice and vegetables, which are probably the most delicious and powerful when unadorned. They were simple wholesome foods, holy foods, and we said, "Thank you." To be home again and safe and eating that healing food was a glorious gift.

CHAPTER 9

THE BORDER GUARD

One of the reasons a gap exists between intellect and behavior is that many behaviors are automatic, habitual, and reflexive. They occur without thinking, because the conscious brain is usually too busy with other matters (sometimes loftier, sometimes not) to maintain direct, hands-on control of everything that happens in the body. It would be time-consuming and chaotic if the brain had to maintain conscious control of every sensation coming through every sensory nerve at every instant. There wouldn't be room for anything else on the switchboard if every terrain the feet encounter and every smell the nose detects and every visual image has to come to consciousness.

Instead, the brain delegates certain functions, incorporating them into behaviors we call reflexes or habits. The finger-on-the-flame illustrates this. When the nerve ending in the finger senses the heat from a flame, a message travels along the nerve, first through the finger, then through the hand, wrist, forearm, arm, neck, and finally into the spinal cord. From there, the information heads north, to the brain, which recognizes that there's something hot on the finger, so it might be a good idea to move the finger away from the heat before it burns off. The brain sends a message back down a different nerve to the spinal cord, which eventually gets the message into the arm so that the biceps muscle can jerk up the forearm and pull the finger out of the flame. If it took that long every time, we'd end up with a lot of burned fingers, so the brain let's a spinal reflex handle it, which means that as soon as the message hits the cord, the cord sends the get-the-finger-out message right back, before the brain even knows what's going on. By the time the brain is aware that something was hot, the finger is safely away. It's a quicker, easier, safer, and more efficient way to handle these situations.

This is a beneficial reflex, but unfortunately, many behaviors become reflexive which aren't too helpful. Smokers often tell me that they feel an urge to light a cigarette when they have a cup of coffee. Smelling the familiar aroma and hearing the tinkling in the cup automatically makes them reach for the pack and the lighter. I have one patient who for years stopped in a bakery for donuts on his way to work because he had to pass the shop to get to his office. It became a reflex triggered by the smell of fat and sugar.

The problem is that these potentially harmful reflexes often happen as quickly as the good ones. The brain knows better, but there isn't time to intervene. As it is with the spinal reflex which handles the finger-flame problem, the cigarette is between the lips or the donut is in the mouth before the brain is even aware of what's going on. We need a way to stop the flow of automatic behavior, to buy some time and give the brain a chance to make a specific decision, and not just leave it to a reflex. I've told many patients to hire a border guard, to dream up an imaginary someone, maybe with a funny-looking hat and a badge and a uniform, to stand guard or patrol in front of an imaginary gate that sits in front of the mouth and yell, "Stop! Who goes there?" whenever something wants to get in.

I say to think of the mouth as one of the body's most important borders, where the external environment meets the internal one, and things come and go. Food and air enter, then carbon dioxide and water vapor exit. When too many of the wrong things get in too often - whether it's high-fat food, cigarette smoke, or a virus - it can make you sick sooner or later. I say post a border guard to control the traffic, to regulate what gets in and when, to give the brain a chance to decide what's appropriate and what isn't so that the will has a chance to direct behavior rather than leaving it to habits and reflexes. A border guard allows you to bridge the gap between intellect and behavior, because the guard interrupts the behavior while it consults with the intellect. Most times, when the intellect has an opportunity to decide, it makes the right decision because it usually knows what to do, but first it has to get that opportunity.

I worked with my patient who liked his donuts before work to try and dissect the reflex and insert the border guard at the critical decision point. "You're walking down the street on your way to work and pass the donut shop," I tell him. "Your nose says, 'Boy, that sure smells good.' Your taste buds, awakened by your nose, tell you, 'Let's get some,' and before you know it your feet are involved and they carry you into the shop. Your salivary glands have been alerted by this time and are already dumping watery, enzyme-rich secretions into your mouth. Even your stomach is starting to churn and roll and grind, anticipating what's coming."

"You select and pay quickly while your brain thinks about a work project, an after-work commitment, or something that happened the night before. You start walking out the door, your hand already in the bag feeling the soft, cool powdered sugar. The donut comes out and up to your mouth, but then something happens. A voice shouts, 'Stop! Who goes there?' It's tough luck for your nose and mouth and stomach as it appears the border guard is on duty. Your hands and nose and eyes say, 'It's donuts, sir.' 'Donuts, eh,' the guard says; 'Let's see your papers.'"

"The border guard summons the brain, bringing it back from wherever it was, and announces, 'Donuts, requesting passage. The nose found them, the tongue asked for them, and now the stomach wants them, too.' The brain examines things carefully, then speaks: 'Donuts, you say; you mean powdered sugar, shortening, a little refined bleached white flour, more sugar, cream, and all of it deep-fried, right? I'm afraid not. Everyone received the memo last Monday about us being in the diet-mode, remember? We have to lower cholesterol, lose weight, and all of that. Now as I recall, we attended a wedding reception yesterday. My records show that we had dessert

- some kind of whipped, creamy, parfait-type thing. I let that one go, because it was a special occasion. Then some cake was wrapped up to take home, but never made it because it was eaten in the car on the way since it was such a long ride. I let that go, too. We're supposed to be back on track today. These donuts, while not evil in and of themselves, are definitely a bad idea at this time.' 'That's all I needed to hear,' the border guard says. 'Admission DENIED!' The donut goes back into the bag.

In the early 1980's, Dr. Carl Simonton's book *Getting Well Again* tried to help cancer patients visualize a strong immune system utilizing a imaginary inner guide. The patients I see with diet-related health concerns such as heart disease and diabetes can benefit from a similar friend, something which can which embody and give voice to their will.

Eventually, after going through the exercise enough times and having the border guard prevent enough inappropriate entries, people can build some new and more beneficial habits. I have some patients who get to know what the border guard will say before they even try to get something across. At that point they can let go of the guard, because they will have re-discovered and re-created good behavior, and in so doing will re-discover and re-create good health.

CHAPTER 10

WHAT MOTHER RECOGNIZES

In a television commercial advertising margarine in the 1970's, a woman dressed in a long white, flowing gown walked through a forest. Some gentle woodland creatures were nearby - a fawn and a bunny as I recall - and birds were twittering sweetly in the trees. Someone off-screen offered the woman something to eat which looked like a piece of buttered bread. A voice asked her what was on the bread. She dipped her pinky finger into the spread and said, smiling, "That's my butter," implying that she would know it anywhere. "No," the voice told her, "not butter, margarine." First she was incredulous. Then she became angry. "It's not nice to fool Mother Nature," she said through clenched teeth, then raised her arms as thunder sounded, the animals scampered off, the birds stopped singing, and one blissful, bucolic scene turned a little ugly.

I suppose the commercial was clever. The manufacturer and the ad agency wanted people to imagine a margarine so good and butter-like that even Mother Nature could be fooled. When you think about it, though, it was probably inaccurate, and also a little perverted. If a real Mother Nature existed, I don't think she would have been duped. I imagine she would have said, scowling, "What is this? I know it looks a little like butter (although the color is not quite right), and it feels a little like butter (although the consistency is not quite right), but the taste... this is definitely not butter."

When this commercial was made Americans were starting to understand the relationship between saturated fats and heart disease. I remember caring for heart attack patients during my training and how glum they looked in their hospital beds after meeting with the dietitian and learning they had to substitute vegetable oils and margarine for butter. I heard their gastronomic distress repeatedly, since they preferred to spread butter on their toast, or plop it like a brick on their pancakes, or use it to drown their green vegetables. I even heard some people complain that margarine reminded them of wartime rationing, which didn't fit with their perception of American prosperity.

I suppose one group must have been happy about the news - margarine manufacturers. If butter was bad, they could give us something safer to spread and plop and melt on stuff. "Rich in poly-unsaturates" was another familiar phrase used to sell the butter-wanna-be's and their close cousins, the cooking and salad oils. We've found out more recently that margarine may not be so good after all, since it's high in something called "trans fatty acids" formed when they hydrogenate the vegetable oils so they will be solid at room temperature and resemble butter. These trans acids may be just as prone to clog arteries as the saturated fats in the real stuff, which lead the Washington, DC-based Center for Science in the Public Interest (CSPI) to ask the FDA to include them with the saturated fats on food labels (see the April, 1994 issue of CSPI's *Nutrition Action Healthletter*). I chuckled when I read this, because my imaginary Mother Nature could have told us to avoid margarine without knowing any organic chemistry or performing any chemical testing. Right after she said, "This is definitely not butter" we could have asked her it was safer. She would have probably said, "If you make it look like butter, and make it feel like butter, and even try (unsuccessfully) to make it taste like butter, what in the world makes you think for even a minute that it won't affect your body the way butter does?"

I had my right brain Mother Nature in mind about ten years ago while attending a picnic. A pleasant woman offered me a dessert -

some kind of green gelled thing with a white and creamy substance spread over the top which the label called a non-dairy whipped topping. She said, "It's low-cal." When I asked what that meant she explained that the dessert had close to zero calories. I'm a little mellower these days, so if the same thing happened now I would probably simply say, "No, thank you," and drop it. But I was a contentious son-of-a-gun back then, always itching for a dietary scuffle, so I snapped back, "No calories, eh? Then it must not contain any food either; unless, of course, you're offering me water, which is the only calorie-free substance I know is safe to consume." Ironically, she had innocently offered me the dish because she had heard I was "into nutrition" and therefore assumed I would appreciate something low in calories. She looked a little bemused, even hurt, so said as calmly as I could, "Food has calories, so no calories means it's not food."

I realized that my imaginary Mother Nature was speaking, and decided to judge food the way Mother Nature would and eat only what she recognizes. If the food has been so altered that even its own Mother doesn't recognize it, maybe we should avoid it. Although it's dualistic to say "Never", it's okay to say "Not often". A few months later I had a chance to apply this principle in one of my medical school lectures. A student asked me what was wrong with saccharin, the leading artificial sweetener of the day (before aspartame). He asked if I didn't like the substance because it had been associated with bladder cancer in laboratory animals. "Not really," I said, "the animal doses were huge, and the results may not be applicable to humans." I told him that my objection was much simpler and more basic. "It's made from coal tar," I said, "and coal tar isn't food."

I began having imaginary dialogues with Mother. Here's what I thought might happen if I offered her a piece of white bread:

- Here, Mother, try some bread.
- Bread? You call this bread? What is it made from?
- Wheat, Mother. What else?

- Wheat? Wheat, you say? The wheat I make is brown. This "bread" is white.
- Oh, that. We took out the brown parts. They were kind of coarse and unrefined.
- Oh you did, did you? What you call the "brown parts" were the germ and the bran   and they happen to be very important. I wouldn't have put them in there if I thought they could be left out. Oh my poor, poor wheat, what have they done to you?
- We thought it would make it better. Lighter. Fluffier. Not so rough.
- This stuff is light, all right; so light it could probably float away. And fluffy, you've got that right. I could squeeze this into a ball and bounce it down the street. This isn't bread. Don't call it "bread". Call it "baked aerated raped flour", but don't insult me and dishonor my precious wheat by calling it "bread".

My Mother Nature has a good time in the supermarket these days, checking out the limp, beat, overcooked stuff in cans that's supposed to be vegetables, or trying to figure out why the "fruit snacks" contain no fruit. No, it isn't nice to fool Mother Nature. Actually, it's not even nice to try. In the television commercial, the punishment was thunder and lightning and rain, but in real life, we pay a much higher price—heart attack, diabetic amputations, colon cancer, and premature death.

But forget for a minute about diet-related illnesses and all the depressing statistics about heart disease and stroke and cancer. I see another more fundamental reason why we shouldn't try to fool Mother. I consider it disrespectful and almost un-American. Some of our holidays and clichés suggest that we have a special place in our hearts for mothers. We talk about the flag and apple pie and Mom. We think about mothers especially in the month of May when we buy greeting cards and send flowers and create a holiday in their honor. This is nothing new or simply the creation of greeting card and flower association lobbying efforts, because many ancient peoples paid homage to Mother in May, too - our Mother, the Earth. Very old May Day rituals celebrated the fertility and fecundity of our planet, which was often thought of as a Mother, married, in a way, to Father Sky.

I think about Mother Nature as the source of all food and all life, and feel she is alive in so much of what we see, hear, feel, taste, and smell. I particularly think about smells in May, Mother's month, and remember how acute that sense is in children. I read an article in a magazine once which said that infants, whom we presume don't see all that well, can recognize their mothers and pick them out of a pack, just by their smell. So many of my own childhood memories ride on smells. When I walk around outside in May, with all the wonderful fragrances around, so much from my boy-years comes back: the smells of lilacs, azaleas, fresh cut wet lush spring grass, warm breezes, and the unmistakable scent of spring rain.

I smell the sweat of children, that mildly sweet pre-pubescent smell. It's on my children after they've been running around in the warm May evening, when their mother calls them in for dinner. I remember the same smell on my brothers and friends, and I can hear my own mother's voice singing out over the backyards and into the gathering dusk, calling us in to eat. I remember the same smell on my classmates in the schoolyard at recess time. I smell the flowers now, and I remember the flower wreaths we made in May in my Catholic grade school to crown statues of the Blessed Virgin Mary, whose month, naturally, is May. Our school had a May procession, where we walked around the grounds, two-by-two, hands folded, singing "Immaculate Mary, our hearts are on fire" and "humbly thy children are calling on thee". Singing to Mary, our "lovely Queen of May", who, for Roman Catholics, was the Mother of God, and the symbolic Mother of us all. The smells of the flowers traveled on the heaven-sent breeze that refreshed us and saved us as we stood in line on those hot May afternoons. I smell May flowers now, the perfume of our Mother, the Earth, and I can hear the singing.

I walk outside in the woods today in May and smell the dampness, the richness, and I remember the first girl I ever loved when I was twelve, in sixth grade, and the sweet awakening May woods where we walked to be alone, and barely kissed, lightly, briefly. I smell the woods now, and I can see her and smell her perfume; I can hear our favorite songs. I smell it all today, and I remember everything, instantly, like a flood. They are the smells of our Mother, and the gifts of memory. The smell of her breath on the breeze, and her skin in the ground, and her hair in the flowers and grass. I smell it, and like the blurry-eyed infant, I recognize her.

I think of the food our Mother has prepared for us, the food that grows out of her, the simple roots, leaves, flowers, fruits, and seeds of plants. For many of the patients I counsel, the smells and sights and tastes have become unfamiliar - too coarse, too wild. They don't recognize our Mother, and I correlate the degree of unfamiliarity with how far they have strayed into the processed, altered, adulterated, violated foods our Mother would have never made for us and can't even recognize because we've changed them so much.

I tell them to listen for our Mother calling us over the backyards and into our lengthening journey to tell us to come home for supper. Some of them don't want to come home, and have to be threatened, even punished to get them to come. Every time their bathroom scales give them numbers they can't believe, or their clothes are too tight, or their energy levels are poor, or their bowels don't move, I tell them Mother is calling. Some of them don't hear her calling until they are really hurting with hearts and legs that don't get enough circulation or with cholesterol- polluted blood and cancer-invaded organs. Some don't hear at all, or refuse to come home, or start out too late and die before they get there. But many hear, head for home, and hopefully will get there safely and to stay.

When you can, walk outside in May, or any time. Inhale deeply and recognize our Mother. Hear her voice when the wind moves through the trees. Taste the simple, wholesome meal she prepares for us every day. And the next time you're faced with a food choice or an eating decision, think about Mother. See if you can recognize her in the food, then run it by her in your mind to see if she would recognize it. Imagine what she would say. If she looks at it kind of funny, as if it's unfamiliar, don't even take a chance. If she embraces it as one of her own, as one of her children, eat heartily. Remember, you are one of her children, too, so try to keep things in the family. Eat the foods she would recognize, the foods that let you recognize her, and hopefully she will continue to recognize you.

$$\boxed{\text{CHAPTER 11}}$$

THE DIET JUNGLE

Many of my patients balk when I suggest they try a few meatless suppers every week. They seem almost incapable of conceiving a meal without meat, as if there has to be a huge slab of flesh taking up most of the room on the dish or else, hey, it just isn't an official meal. They will tolerate starches and vegetables as side dishes, as satellites orbiting around the star, but not as the main attraction.

When I was growing up in the 1950's and 1960's and asked my mom, "What's for dinner?" she usually answered "Roast Beef" or "Steak" or "Chicken", naming the meal by meat. When Catholics had to avoid meat one day a week, our parish calendar had little pictures of fish on every Friday. If a friend recommends a good restaurant and asks, "What did you have?" the response is often "I had the swordfish" or "I had the surf and turf" or "I had the prime rib", which correlates with the way restaurant menus often list their entrees: Meats; Poultry; Fish.

It's time to make the grains, beans, vegetables and fruits the main part of the meal, and make the flesh the side dish. Many of my patients are trying this already, but frequently tell me they're not exactly sure how much meat to eat. They've read or heard that three to four ounces a serving is appropriate, which was what we told our participants when I worked at the Pritikin Center. People still have problems though, and ask "How much is that?" and "Is it three and a half ounces before cooking or after?" or "Do I actually have to weigh this or can I estimate?" One woman complained to me that she didn't have enough space on her counter for a scale.

I've told many patients to forget scales and rulers and instead to picture their diets as a dense jungle or rainforest, where the first striking is that there's vegetation everywhere - huge tropical leaves, vines hitting them in the face, stalks and stems and tangles so thick they have to cut through with a machete.

But where are the animals in this diet jungle? Real jungles have more life forms than anywhere else on the planet, but sometimes you don't see any animals right away. Maybe you hear them, though, calling to each other or defining their territory, so you conclude they must be in the trees or behind bushes or in the grass.

Now picture your dinner plate and re-create the jungle. You should see lots of green leaves, tangles of roots and beans and grains and fruits. Where's the meat? Where are the animals? Just as it was in the real jungle, hide the meat in your diet jungle, too. Put it in the bushes, buried under leaves, obscured by the vegetation.

When serving meat, bury it under the leaves. Whether it's fish, chicken, or lean red meat, cover it with cabbage or kale or romaine lettuce leaves. I say that if you can readily see the flesh on your plate, you're eating too much, and that it's better if you have to look around for it, dig a little, and finally uncover it under some vegetables.

Get the eye used to seeing something different on the plate. Feel right at home with dense vegetation, the more the better. Don't feel comfortable without a huge mound of rice or pasta, or a monstrous pile of vegetables. Be surprised when you find a small serving of meat, either by itself or cut into small pieces and scattered through the other foods; pleasantly surprised if you're so inclined, but know that you didn't necessarily have to have it, that it still would have been a satisfying and nourishing meal without it.

Don't let your diet jungle frighten you. You'll be safe as long as the animals stay hidden. And the next time you wonder how much meat to eat, remember this: eat as much meat as you can't see on the plate. That's probably just enough.

CHAPTER 12

HUNGER IS A BANK ACCOUNT OF FIRE

The procession of Dakota Sioux which begins Ruth Beebe Hill's novel *Hanta Yo* says that the second place in line was reserved for "the one who carries the smoldering wood, the source of a cooking fire." This important, almost legendary tribal role of "keeper of the flame" originally meant a literal tending, protecting, and carrying fire, which provided heat, energy for cooking, a tool to keep away predatory animals, and brought light into darkness. Fire meant life for pre-industrial cultures, so they had to maintain it and never let it go out. It has since become a metaphor for any individual or institution charged with preserving or protecting the vitality of something precious.

The hunger that's like a fire in the belly should never go out either. It's as precious as real fire was, so you can't let it disappear. You should never eat to fullness or be completely satisfied after a meal. Being stuffed and loosening the belt means that you've extinguished the hunger fire, doused it with gluttony. So leave the table before you're full, as if you were leaving with a credit. Don't spend all your hunger at one time. Think of it as a bank account of fire. Use it when you need to, but always save a little bit, always leave something in the account. Keep the flame alive. Let that smoldering hunger strengthen and intensify so it can drive you to your next meal. You'll have the security of knowing you have something left over, something extra. When you overeat beyond hunger, you have to replenish the account because you withdrew too much. It's always more comfortable knowing you have a little something put away.

Chronically needing to pay back is a tough way to live. Some people play the game of chasing their overeating with exercise, perennially trying and usually failing to burn off their excesses. One patient even admitted that, "I exercise so I can eat more." He would add up his excess calories, then determine from an exercise physiology chart how much he'd have to run to maintain equilibrium. Every day I examine someone who tells me he or she is overweight because of a lack of exercise, not even mentioning the need to eat less because, "I really don't eat that much." Most times they're deluding themselves, unless they plan to be exercise maniacs who will run, walk, bike, or swim miles and miles every day and generate enormous calorie deficits. Otherwise, it doesn't work because there's such a huge disparity between what you can burn from exercise and what you accumulate from eating. It's a gross mismatch. My patients already know how easy it is to put it on, and how hard to take it off.

When you leave the table with a hunger credit, you create an energy debit. The energy you didn't take in has to be paid out of your savings account (stored fat). It's simple accounting. Every pound of fat contains about 3500 calories. To gain a pound of fat you have to eat 3500 calories which don't get burned, 3500 calories beyond your metabolic needs. You can do this by eating 100 extra calories every day for 35 days, which is very easy to do with a couple of cookies, a piece and a half of dry toast, six ounces of apple juice, or ten pieces of gum. One hundred extra calories a day is an easy pound every 35 days, and a little over ten pounds a year. It adds up.

When you accumulate hunger credits and get daily energy debits of 100 calories, you lose a pound of fat every 35 days and ten pounds a year. These add up, too. As I said, it's simple accounting.

It's okay to spend your credits once in a while - on your birthday, vacations, holidays, and other special occasions. Don't hoard them obsessively, but don't spend them all, either. Always save a few. Always stay a little hungry. Tend your fire. Keep it going. Let its warmth and brightness wash over you, keeping you alive.

$$\boxed{\text{CHAPTER 13}}$$

THE WEDDING RECEPTION - 1983

Kathy and I were guests at a friend's wedding where they served a sit-down dinner at the reception. It was three-thirty in the afternoon and we hadn't eaten since breakfast so we were starved. The appetizer was a fruit cup that looked pretty lame. I tasted it, but that was all, since it was obviously out of a jar, sickeningly sweet in heavy syrup, and not too appetizing.

The salad came next, and was actually pretty good with a mix of romaine and some other dark greens (crisp, and possibly local since it was early summer) with grated carrots, chickpeas, a slice of canned beet, and a creamy Italian dressing. The dressing was a little oily, and I doubt that it had any olive oil, but I ate it all.

The main course was pretty predictable banquet fare for this part of the world - stuffed capon, baked potato, and string beans almandine. We stopped eating fowl in 1979, but Kathy had started again in 1982 when she was pregnant. While she was breastfeeding (which she was at the time) she would eat just about anything she could get her hands on. I warned her, tongue-in-cheek, that I thought I could smell hormone and antibiotic residues in the capon. She told me I was crazy and cleaned her plate. God bless her.

I passed on the bird, but ate all of the baked potato (including the skin) without the available butter or sour cream. "Isn't that awfully dry?" someone at the table asked me. "Not when you chew it a hundred times," I replied, "that's why God created saliva." The string beans and slivered almonds were pretty greasy, but I ate all mine as well as the portions from four others at our table. "It's vegetables and nuts," I kept telling myself, trying to ignore the little oil spill on the plate.

Dessert was a frozen parfait with a red swirl, the color of which I have never seen in any food that grows, walks, or swims. Mine melted untouched while I was on the dance floor doing the Bunny Hop. I refused the wedding cake, too, but Kathy took her piece home. A month later, we found it in the refrigerator, looking as good (or as bad) as the day we brought it home. "Want some?" she offered. "No thanks," I told her, "I won't eat food so protected against spoilage that it could survive a thermonuclear explosion." She gave me her what-am-I-going-to-do-with-him look and shook her head as she licked a fingerful of icing before tossing it.

CHAPTER 14

CALIBRATING THE TONGUE

I think of the tongue as a taste-o-meter, a recording instrument. Natural and man-made chemicals in foods and other substances interact with specialized tongue-tissues called taste buds, then send messages to the brain which we eventually interpret as taste or flavor. All recording instruments need calibration An unmarked thermometer can be stuck into a pot of boiling water, then marked as the boiling point where the mercury stops rising. A device for recording music needs to have an instrument which will pick up the highs and lows or else the piece will play back unbalanced. It won't sound right. It won't be pleasant. It won't accomplish what the composer intended.

It's the same with food, where the wide spectrum of flavors and textures demands a tongue which is calibrated to sense and record them all, or the diet might be unbalanced. I believe our tongues need serious re-calibration, which I attribute to several decades of eating the processed, refined, high-fat, high-salt, high-sugar foods that have jaded our palates. To find our eating way home we must learn to appreciate the simple, subtle flavors in natural, unadulterated foods. This means teaching the tongue new definitions of sweet, rich, and salty, which can't just be a sensory exercise, since the new flavors will be too bland for our desensitized taste buds. There has to be a cognitive or thinking component, too. The brain, which knows all the health reasons for changing the diet, has to encourage the tongue with the justifications for accommodating to the new foods, or the tongue will never buy into it.

Let me illustrate this by telling what happened the first time I cooked and ate whole grain brown rice. I had grown up eating the white stuff, usually laced with butter or a sauce of some sort. This time I was going for the unrefined brown stuff straight up, because the blurb on the package promised it would be wonderful. First, though, I had an imaginary conversation with my brain.

> **Me** - Hi, brain. It's me. Listen, I'll be sending something new over the tongue at dinner tonight. It's called brown rice. The package speaks glowingly of this stuff; says it's supposed to taste "nutty and sweet". Let me know what you think.
>
> (minutes later, a mouthful goes in, gets chewed quickly, then swallowed)
>
> **Me** - Well? What did you think?
>
> **Brain** - Brown rice, you say?
>
> **Me** - That's right.
>
> **Brain** - Okay, let's see, signals starting to come in from the tongue. Texture: uh, uh, chewy. Very chewy. I'll make a note to keep it between the teeth a little longer next time.
>
> **Me** - What about the flavor? Are you reading "nutty and sweet"?
>
> **Brain** - Checking. I'm checking. Going through the files. Under "nutty" we have things like smoked, salted, sugared almonds, walnuts, pecans. Now cross-matching. Uh, sorry, this rice isn't anything like that, so I can't call it "nutty".
>
> **Me** - What about "sweet"? Are you picking up anything there?
>
> **Brain** - Checking that right now. Okay. Let me put it this way: it's not like anything sweet that you're used to eating.
>
> **Me** - Well, brain, here's how it is: we're changing the way we eat around here. Starting a new life and all that.
>
> **Brain** - It isn't day-after-New-Year's, is it?

Me - No. Now stop and listen. This isn't some fly-by-night program or a post-holiday- guilt thing. This is for real. This will be forever.

Brain - Interesting.

Me - Anyway, foods such as this brown rice will figure prominently in the new order of things, so I think it would help if we liked it. It's supposed to be very good for us, and there may be other foods like it that we need to get to like, too.

Brain - I'll see what I can do. I'll get with the tongue, have my people talk to his   people. We'll set up a meeting.

(several days later, we try again with another serving of brown rice)

Brain - Brown rice, again?

Me - Yep. What do you think.

Brain - Actually, I have some good news for you/us. After our last experiment I got some very good reports from a lot of different areas about this stuff. The bowels definitely like it. Some fat deposits inside the arteries actually started to shrink and blood is getting into places it hasn't been in years. And wait until you hear this: I had a long talk with the tongue, and last night we were up late working on the taste buds, re-calibrating. We re-set them for MAX sensitivity, and guess what just came up on the screen? Nutty and sweet!

After you've re-calibrated your tongue, it can guide you as a back-up to your border guard. It will take something you used to call sweet and tell you it is sickeningly sweet. This happened to me recently when I was standing on the sidelines at my older daughter's soccer game. One of the other parents had made chocolate brownies as an after-game treat and was passing around extras to the other moms and dads. When the plastic container came my way I declined. The dad said, jokingly I think, "What, you'd insult me by not eating one of my wife's brownies?" I was a little embarrassed, so I took one and bit into it in front of him. "Mmm," I said, "Very tasty." Actually it was much too tasty, sweeter and richer than anything I had eaten in years, and I couldn't finish it.

What used to be deliciously rich will become grotesquely greasy, as when I inadvertently ate a piece of chicken skin at a barbecue. And what used to be perfectly seasoned will become intolerably salty, which is how I find the usual movie theater popcorn. With a re-calibrated tongue, a carrot will become sweet, while an over-ripe pear becomes almost too sweet. A bowl of bean stew will become rich and hearty, and a simple stalk of celery will become satisfyingly salty. And, who knows, if you make the right adjustments on the tongue, a mouthful of brown rice will become you know what.

CHAPTER 15

EATING MY CROSS

S ince I was an English major in college I have a particular interest in the origin and fate of words. I often wonder what happened to the word diet. I've heard it used to refer generically to a certain group's or culture's way of eating, as when a textbook or a television documentary discusses the diet of the Aztecs or the diet of the Inuit people. When my patients use the word it usually means penance and represents suffering. It's something painful and unpleasant they put off for painful, unpleasant days such as Mondays or the first day back from vacation or the day after a holiday. It is payment for the committed sins of over-indulgence and poor self-control, or the inherited sins from grandparents, the metabolic-baggage-cliché-curse that converts the sight-of-food into stored fat.

Diet has become a cross for many of the people I counsel, a symbol of suffering like the one Jesus carried and invited his followers to "take up" when he said that, to follow him, you had to "take up your cross". Carrying the cross has become a metaphor for any excess load, as when people refer to a difficult job or a marital problem as their cross to bear. The diet-cross is a burden that many of my patients pick up at least once in a lifetime, if not three or four times a year or even perennially, weighing them down, causing them to fall. But a cross is a shape, too, and one of our most important food families gets its name from this word. The official name for cabbage family vegetables is *cruciferous*. The word comes from the Latin *crux* which means *cross,* so-named because the first four leaves that sprout form a small cross. Since the word crucifix has the same root, I think of these as the cross vegetables..

Leafy vegetables in this family include cabbages, Brussels sprouts, broccoli, kale, collard greens, mustard greens, turnip greens, cauliflower, kohlrabi, and others. Cruciferous greens may be some of the best choices in the general category of leafy vegetables. In addition to respectable amounts of calcium and the anti-oxidants Vitamin C and beta-carotene, scientists have recently discovered potentially cancer-preventing chemicals in these foods - compounds with names like indoles and isothiocyanates. All these beneficial components may at least partly explain why people who frequently eat these foods tend to get fewer cancers overall according to Dr. John Potter at the University of Minnesota's Cancer Prevention Center (interviewed in the April, 1994 issue of the Center for Science in the Public Interest's *Nutrition Action Healthletter*).

This means that we should eat vegetables from this group several times a week, if not daily. It means that while lettuce, string beans, spinach, and peas are fine foods, I don't feel I've eaten all the green vegetables I need until I've had kale or collards or cabbage, too.

Think of your diet as the flexible way you always eat rather than something you go *on* on Mondays, only to go *off* on Fridays. Don't make it a burdensome cross, but a leafy one, a cross you can eat instead of carry. Eat cross-vegetables and you'll carry your cross inside you, but instead of weighing you down or making you fall, it will strengthen you and lighten your load.

CHAPTER 16

THANKSGIVING WEEKEND - 1986

THURSDAY

I told my three-and-a-half year-old daughter Elizabeth that the people in England were mean to the Pilgrims so they hopped on the Mayflower and came to America which wasn't yet called America. She wanted to know how and why they were mean, because they seemed perfectly nice and civilized when she watched Prince Andrew's wedding on television. And didn't we wave to the people in England last summer when we looked out over the Atlantic Ocean from the top of the Ferris wheel on the Ocean City, New Jersey Boardwalk? I told her that the people who were mean to the Pilgrims lived a long time ago, before her and before me and Mommy and before Prince Andrew and before the Ocean City boardwalk.

I really didn't want to discuss religious persecution with a toddler, so I distracted Elizabeth by enlisting her help in the kitchen. Kathy and I had taken the huge step of inviting some family to our house for Thanksgiving dinner, which meant that for the very first time ever, our kitchen and by extension our whole house would have the aroma of a roasting turkey. We purchased the bird from a local farmers' market where a Pennsylvania Dutch family had a poultry concession. They assured us that their birds roamed free and weren't fed hormones or antibiotics. Kathy handled the turkey, and other family members had been assigned to bring assorted side dishes and desserts. I decided to make a few things which I had read or imagined the Pilgrims and Indians must have eaten, with a few modern innovations. It was a big project, but with Elizabeth's help it only took twice as long.

I started with what the Lenni Lenape Indians of southeastern Pennsylvania referred to as the *three sisters*: corn, beans, and squash. The corn bread had stone-ground whole grain yellow corn meal, whole wheat pastry flour, soymilk, cold pressed corn oil (I use canola today, but it wasn't around at the time), and aluminum-free baking powder. The beans were limas, soaked and then boiled with dried corn to make the Indian dish succotash. Then there was the squash pie, a vegetable side dish made only with pureed butternut squash and diced onions which is naturally sweet. I also made some cranberry sauce by boiling the berries with apple and pear chunks, mashing it with a potato masher, and thickening it with some agar - a seaweed gelling agent. I sweetened it with maple syrup, but must have used too much because everyone thought it tasted great.

My contribution to dessert was a pumpkin pie, adapted from a recipe I had found years ago on the label from some canned pumpkin. I pureed boiled pumpkin (actually the canned variety is fine, too) using a hand-mill in an attempt to burn my own calories instead of fossil fuels, soymilk instead of condensed cow's milk, egg whites instead of whole eggs (from those same clean-living poultry farmers), then cinnamon, ginger, and cloves. Maple syrup was my sweetener instead of white and brown sugar, once again keeping with the New England theme, and I baked the whole thing in a rather heavy corn oil and whole wheat pastry flour crust. While I liked it fine, it didn't go over with the rest of the crowd as well as the cranberry sauce (maybe not enough syrup).

It was some feast. The golden cornbread, the orange squash pie, the red cranberries, the brown pumpkin, and the various greens and yellows everyone else brought were a delight for the eye as well as the taste buds. Then came the moment of decision for me. Everyone waited to see what I would do, knowing I hadn't eaten any animal flesh in over seven years. "Will he eat any turkey?" they wondered. "Can he resist?"

I hadn't had any trouble avoiding meat prior to that, but it was definitely tougher that year after smelling the bird cooking all day. I expected to be repulsed by it; but was surprised to find it strangely alluring. Finally I tasted a piece. Then another. It was delicious.

FRIDAY

Uncharacteristically, I took a holiday the day after Thanksgiving that year. The four-day weekend made me feel like a schoolboy again, and I learned that when you don't have to work for four days in a row, the word thanksgiving takes on a new meaning.

I decided to indulge myself and do nothing all day. The day before had been an exhausting cooking marathon followed by an all-night clean-up, so I had no guilt about my decision to loaf. I didn't read, think, or do any chores. My goal was to move as little as possible, but I took passivity one step further and sat in front of the television most of the morning. I couldn't remember the last time I had been home on a weekday, and noted an entirely different feel than a weekend day. I hadn't watched weekday television in a long time, either, and found the interview shows and info-mercials so boring that I made about ten trips into the kitchen, opening every cabinet door and the refrigerator each time, looking for something to eat (I didn't know at the time how to unmask the masquerader).

Then around noon, the TV screen came alive with sitcom reruns from the fifties and sixties. Not only could I watch Dick Van Dyke, Andy Griffith, and *Leave It to Beaver* one after another, but I also got my inspiration for lunch, since every kid in sitcom land was eating peanut butter sandwiches that day. I made my way to the kitchen for the eleventh time, but with the mission to make the definitive P.B. & J - a peanut butter and jelly sandwich. It was the lunch that won my childhood heart and fueled the boomers when they were babies. However, I made and ate the new and improved 1980's version of the classic, the one that could safely fulfill my sentimental and gustatory needs.

The peanut butter was one made from roasted peanuts only - no salt, sugar, added fats. The peanuts had been certified aflatoxin-free, the bread was whole grain, of course, not the white fluffy stuff the kids on T.V. were tossing down, and the jelly was made from only grapes and grape juice with pectin. I assembled it as quickly as I could, but before sinking in my teeth, I completed a ritual, holy and ceremonious act. I licked the knife.

Rhythm

CHAPTER 17

WHAT GEESE KNOW

Summer's end first becomes noticeable in August here in
southeastern Pennsylvania. It still gets very hot and humid, but
not the way it does in July. The leaves are still green, but it's a paler
shade, and some yellow and brown ones have already dropped by late
in the month when they rattle under lawnmowers and float on top of
the neighborhood swim club pool where the water is too cold for
swimming until well after noon.

Late in August you might even see the season's first skein of
Canada geese, honking into town from who-knows-where up north in
their characteristic V-formation. It means that Arctic winds are
kicking up wherever these geese had just been. While I may find it
hard to think about winter in summer, these geese are already
responding to it.

What makes geese pick up and go? I've often wondered about
this. Is it the shortening day or the first gust of polar air and a subtle
drop in temperature? Could it be a change in the angle of sunlight as
the earth moves subtly, or a somewhat smaller food supply? What do
geese see or hear or feel that stirs them to flight?

What do geese know?

What they know is that their death is coming with winter,
speaking in August's cooler air and saying, "Stay where you are,
keep doing what you're doing, and I'll take you. Soon." So they

answer. With a flurry of honks and flapping wings they say, "No, not soon. It will have to be later. We're taking off."

When patients sit in my office and ask for help with their diets, I wonder what has inspired them to change. What makes them pick up and go, leaving the way they used to eat and looking for something better, safer? Some say very specifically that they need to lower cholesterol, lose weight; prevent the colon cancer a parent had, or control blood pressure or diabetes without medication. Others are more general and say they want to look and feel better or have more energy. These are all good answers, but I sense something beneath all their concrete reasons, as with the forty-three year-old advertising executive Ron with high blood pressure and high cholesterol who told me at his initial visit that his father had the same risk factors and died of a heart attack at age fifty-two. For the first time he realized he might be on the same track. He had never thought about death before, but now he could see his mortality on the lab slip, or hear it in my voice after I reported what I'd heard through my stethoscope. He recalled the Don Juan books by Carlos Castaneda, and how the sorcerer used to say that death was always lurking over our left shoulders, stalking us, waiting to take us, forcing us to live differently. Ron had struggled twenty years with thirty excess pounds, but vowed that day to change his diet permanently.

I see death tease people when it gets close enough to grab their hearts or squeeze their legs and scare them, but not kill them. I give their symptoms formal, clinical names such as angina or claudication, but it's really death, taking a swipe and saying, "Stay where you are, keep doing what you're doing, and I'll take you. Soon." I see it corrode their bones and sweeten their blood and call it arthritis or diabetes but it's death saying, "Stay where you are, keep doing what you're doing, and I'll take you. Soon." I see it put lumps in women's breasts or inside men's bowels and the surgeons and pathologists call it tumor or carcinoma but it's death saying, "Stay where you are, keep doing what you're doing, and I'll take you. Soon."

The problem with soon is that it's often too soon, too early. No one avoids death forever, but I practice Preventive Medicine and try to follow my own advice because I believe that premature death is avoidable. I was counseling a sixty-four year-old maintenance worker recently whom I had just diagnosed with diabetes. I was explaining how important it was to get this problem under control with diet and exercise because of what diabetes can do to the circulation, the kidneys, the eyes, the peripheral nervous system, and how it increased his risk for heart attack. I may have overwhelmed him somewhat, because he chuckled and said, "Well, Doc, when your number's up there isn't a whole lot you can do about it." But I told him that his number didn't have to be up yet, and that even though death would eventually come calling, he didn't have to invite it in ahead of schedule.

I want us to know how to answer when death speaks prematurely. I want us to honk and flap our wings at death, to hiss at it with the steam from our pots of brown rice and beans and say, "No, not soon. It will have to be later." We need to know what geese know, to be able to see and feel death, to listen to it, to let it get us up and going.

If you ever hear death speak to you, saying it wants to take you soon, shake the rinsing water off a couple of cabbage leaves and pretend you're flapping your wings. Let the rhythmic vegetable chopping on a cutting board be your honking and say, "I'm taking off."

$$\boxed{\text{CHAPTER 18}}$$

THE SAFE SIDE OF SCARCITY

I had a college Anthropology professor who told our class that Nature abhors a surplus. He was discussing the significance of the switch from hunting and gathering to agriculture as the major means for humans to get food, and how it created problems when one group wanted the stored supplies of another. I found this remarkable, since I had previously heard that Nature abhors a vacuum, that it will always fill up emptiness with something, as when the Big Bang filled the vacuum of space with stars, planets, and energy. But, according to this Anthrologist, Nature also hates fullness and will always do something to move it back toward emptiness.

As I've thought about that lesson over the years, it occurred to me that one of our greatest achievements as a species - our ability to store excess energy and nutrients against hard times or an uncertain food supply - also has a downside, since anything stored is fair game for plunder. If you have surplus, some have-not may eventually try to take it from you, which explains why I occasionally find weevils or worms in my rice, mold on my peaches, ants on a picnic blanket, and mouse droppings by a torn bag of bird seed. Sometimes the have-not has two legs, as when a hungry Jean Valjean in *Les Miserables* stole a loaf of bread.

I've seen Nature abhor a surplus on a much more personal level when my patients eat more than they need and store the what they don't need around their waists and in their arteries. In my right brain moments I see this as another way that Nature attacks excess, since these people with too much storage may prematurely return to the earth where all surplus is consumed.

Humans were programmed a long time ago for scarcity, descended from people whose bodies adapted to make a little bit go a long way. Otherwise, our species would have never survived the inconsistencies in food availability from famines, droughts, and floods, the need to follow migratory animals, or depend on seasonal plants. The genetic adaptation to scarcity is sometimes called the thrifty genotype, an inherited metabolism which stores energy very efficiently because it believes it cannot rely on a consistent supply of food. I've seen this mechanism at work many times when patients try to lose weight on diets providing fewer than a thousand daily calories. They frequently fail because their metabolic rates drop as they shift into the hoarding mode. You need to burn calories to lose weight, but your body won't let you burn them if it thinks you're starving.

The thrifty genotype means that many of us are food-storing machines, which was life-saving before modern times. The dilemma today arises when we place this scarcity programming into a food-abundant environment where it stores and stores and stores against hard times that never come. The result is over-storage, which explodes over belt buckles or implodes inside blood vessels. What makes this worse is that we're not physically active enough to burn off the excess, since we don't chase mammoths across the savanna or flee pursuing saber-toothed tigers any more.

I pretend there may not be enough food tomorrow if I gorge today, that I need to ration a little. I recall that when Europeans rationed during World War Two and had less meat and sugar because of blockades, there was less Heart Disease and Cancer, a trend which reversed when happy days came again. I imagine myself a Paleolithic hunter-gatherer, living most days on the seeds, leaves, and berries we gathered in the fields and woods, with the occasional meat feast after the hunt. Scarcity is always a threat, but I see us as just getting by, always skirting just on the safe side of that line.

If you get used to just enough, too much will feel terrible. Scale everything back. Re-calibrate your storage tanks and adjust the gauge to read "stuffed" at half the previous quantity. Remember that if you're always a full picnic basket, you can be sure the ants will come.

$$\boxed{\text{CHAPTER 19}}$$

BLOTCHED BAGS AND STAINED NAPKINS

As a poor struggling medical student I drove a junker car - a virtually indestructible 1966 Pontiac. It wasn't pretty or stylish or even very clean, but it was affordable transportation with a great heater. To save money, I did some of my own maintenance with a popular book to guide me through such basics as oil and oil filter changes. The book suggested that I could detect oil and other fluid leaks by putting an old sheet or a large piece of cardboard under the car when it was parked overnight, then examine the sheet or board the next day and try to tell by the location of any stains what was leaking and how much. I was able to diagnose an oil leak this way, after which I brought the car to an auto mechanic who confirmed my conclusion with a paternalistic, head-shaking, "Doesn't look good, she's leaking oil."

A few years later I applied the same technique when trying to determine a food's fat content. I could have read the label, consulted a chart in a textbook, or written to the food manufacturer or processor. But it's easier, more immediate, and more tangible to examine the bag the food came in, or to put a napkin under it for several minutes. If I see greasy blotches on the bag, or shiny stains on the serviette, I shake my head and say, "Doesn't look good, she's leaking oil."

While I never say "never", I try to avoid such foods in my diet, or at worst to save them for special occasions and keep the quantity low. There are plenty of other uses for these items, though, such as lubricating noisy hinges and rusty gates, or after a bath to moisturize dry skin, rubbed onto faces and legs for a smooth shave, or even to wax down skis and surfboards. I don't want to eat something too frequently if the fat comes out to get me right through the bag.

CHAPTER 20

NOT COW, LIKE COW (THE CHEWING FOUR-FER)

In his book *Indians in Pennsylvania* Paul A. W. Wallace writes that "Indian corn", or maize, has been called the mother of civilization in America." The book *American Indians Myths and Legends* contains a lovely creation story from the Penobscot Indians called Corn Mother. In it, a goddess named First Mother sacrifices her body so that the earth could be "covered with tall, green, tasseled plants. The plants' fruit – corn – was First Mother's flesh, given so that the people might live and flourish."

After eighteen years of talking to patients about their diets along with casual observations at restaurants, parties, and supermarkets, I've concluded that the major food-god in America is currently the cow. Beef and dairy products have been central items in the American diet for most of this century, although it was probably something of an accident. In the early 1900's fledgling nutritional scientists were trying to describe the optimal human diet and getting very excited about protein and newly discovered B-vitamins as a way to treat and prevent malnutrition. The government saw a way to support beef and dairy farmers and better nourish the population at the same time by promoting these products to the American people. It seemed like a win-win, to insure markets for a growing industry and make sure the consumers would benefit, too. But right after World War II the patterns of disease incidence changed, with infectious diseases such as tuberculosis and bacterial pneumonia on the way out (the result of Public Health improvements in sanitation and housing, and the introduction of antibiotics and immunizations), and problems such as heart attack, stroke, and cancer on the rise. I imagine a closed-door meeting between nutritionists and government health officials where they review the statistics then utter a collective "Uh-oh" when they realize that all the foods they had been touting as protective were strongly implicated as killers.

After the "uh-oh" must have come a "Now what do we do?", because it wasn't just small family farmers anymore, but a large and well-organized agribusiness, with huge, powerful special interest dairy associations and beef-producer lobbies. But it was worse than that because, from what I've seen and heard in my practice, people seemed to have internalized the original message and come to believe that meals were somehow lacking or incomplete without something bovine on the table. When I reviewed my patients' diet diaries in the early 1980's I frequently found beef, milk, or cheese at every meal, sometimes all together as a cheeseburger and milkshake. Some advertisers had even thrown housedresses and earrings on animated or cartooned cows, driving the message deep into the cultural psyche that cow is nurturer, cow is healer, cow is mother. There may have been political fallout as well. Senator George McGovern chaired a famous Senate sub-committee in the mid 1970's which produced the landmark report - *Dietary Goals for the United States* - which urged Americans to eat more grains, beans, and vegetables and fewer animal foods. Senator McGovern's home state was South Dakota, a big beef-producer and he lost a re-election bid soon afterwards. Coincidence? Maybe.

Now when I review diaries or take dietary histories I find more poultry and fish and less beef and whole-milk dairy products. The dairy producers are responding by marketing lower-fat and non-fat options which are obvious on any supermarket shelf. Even the beef industry has some leaner varieties, with some range-fed rather than force-fed animals. These innovations are good because these newer items are certainly healthier alternatives, but bad because we never get at the core of the behavior, the original deeply-implanted message which drives us to make these foods the main parts of our diet.

There is no nutritional reason why cow-products have to be central in our American way of eating, and there are a lot of good reasons why they shouldn't. But there is no reason why these foods have to be entirely eliminated from the American diet, either, unless one is allergic, suffers some other idiosyncratic adverse health effects such as indigestion or upper respiratory congestion, or has a moral objection. Vegetarianism is a choice, not a biologic mandate. Since humans are omnivores, we can eat plants and animals, with relatively more meat appropriate in colder regions such as for Arctic hunters. Beef and dairy food can have a place in a sensible diet, but I think that people leading sedentary lives in temperate climates should tweak them to a less prominent place.

I prefer to use the cow as a teacher instead of a dinner, and gain even clearer insights into how and what to eat. My advice is to eat less *of* the cow, and more *like* the cow. Cows are herbivores, pure vegetarians. They eat grass and will do so exclusively unless the farmer decides they might get fatter faster with corn and soybeans. As ruminants they chew and chew, then regurgitate and chew some more, and their intestines are very long to allow ample time and enough surface area for the digestion and absorption of the nutrients. One way to eat like the cow is to eat more like a herbivore. Even though we are omnivores, I tell my patients to emphasize plant-derived foods.

Another way to eat like the cow is to chew thoroughly. If you love bargains and are naturally attracted to deals that say "two-for-one" (a two-fer), thorough chewing is twice as good so I call it a four-fer. It provides four distinct benefits for the price of one activity: better digestion, better taste, an automatic method for eating less quantity, and a relaxing scalp massage.

When you chew thoroughly it helps to physically and chemically break down the food and enhance digestion and absorption. If you leave the food in your mouth and let your teeth work on it, mix it with saliva, grind and moisten it repeatedly, the food will be in a physical form that will be easy for your intestines to absorb. At the risk of abandoning polite conversation, check out your bowel movement sometime to see how well you chew. If you see whole pieces of food, it suggests you could be doing better. Saliva also contains the digestive enzyme amylase, which begins the chemical breakdown of starches in the mouth, before it even reaches the stomach and intestines.

The second benefit is better taste, which is also related to the pre-digestion of starches by amylase. When this enzyme starts to break down the complex carbohydrates, it turns them into simple sugars such as maltose and glucose, which are naturally sweet. If you think food tastes good after three or four chews, wait until you taste it after fifty. I can remember an experiment we did when I was a high school freshman in a course called Introduction to Physical Sciences. We had to chew crackers until they were mush in our mouths. The entire exercise was aimed at experiencing the ability of salivary amylase to turn starch into sugar. We just sat there and chewed and chewed and chewed. We laughed, too, because the whole thing seemed so ridiculous. The teacher kept saying, "Don't swallow, yet, keep chewing," and then at one point finally asked, "Well, do you taste the sweetness?" It was little biased, since he didn't say, "What do you taste?", but I remember being somewhat surprised if not slightly amazed that the mouth-mash had a distinctly sweet flavor.

When my patients learn to chew more thoroughly, they find they automatically eat more slowly, which in turn translates into eating less. When you slow down, you probably won't gulp as much gas-producing air when you eat, either. Try chewing each mouthful only twenty times, and I guarantee it will take you longer to clean your plate, so that when someone calls out, "Seconds?", you will invariably still be working on "Firsts", and hopefully won't have time for another helping.

Finally, thorough chewing is relaxing, not just because it slows you down, but also because one of the muscles involved with chewing is the *Temporalis*. This is a large muscle which fans out over the temple area of your scalp, then attaches to the top of your jaw bone (the mandible). Every time you chew, this muscle moves up and down, actually kind of massaging the temples. Feel it for yourself some time. Put your fingertips lightly on the lower part your temples and feel the muscle move each time your jaw moves. This relaxation actually produces an additional digestive benefit, since it turns on the parasympathetic nervous system which controls the flow of juices from the stomach, intestines, and pancreas. Ever get indigestion from eating too quickly or eating when you were anxious or upset? Try thorough chewing as an antidote. Watch it slow you down and get you into the mellow-mode.

Macrobiotic teacher Michio Kushi has advised in several of his books that we chew each mouthful "thirty to fifty times". I don't feel it matters if it's ten times or ten thousand. The point is to chew as much and as long as you must to liquefy the food, to get it to the point that you can't keep it in your mouth any more because it has already disappeared down your throat.

CHAPTER 21

COMPANY COMING - 1989

Kathy and I had company for dinner one July evening. Since our guests were only casually acquainted with our way of eating, we decided to prepare and serve something that could and would be included in any respectable gourmet restaurant menu. We chose fish since we assumed they would expect some type of meat. It was a filet of some kind of white meat fish (flounder, halibut, or sole) which Kathy marinated in lemon juice, mustard, fresh grated ginger, and tamari soy sauce, then broiled to flaky perfection. Before that, though was my famous (in my house, anyway) squash soup, made by pureeing boiled butternut squash and onions together with a little dill (If the squash sounds a little like my Thanksgiving feast fare, you're right. I should probably write a cookbook called Fifty Uses for Butternut Squash. It has become something of a staple). Everyone marveled at how sweet the soup was, especially since there was no added sweetener.

Along with the fish we had pasta primavera - onions, carrots, yellow summer squash, broccoli, and wild mushrooms sautéed with some extra virgin olive oil and garlic, served over whole wheat fettuccine. Everyone agreed it was delicious, and unable to resist the teaching moment I said, "Isn't it incredible that vegetables actually have a flavor, even without drowning them in butter or a cheese sauce?"

Dessert was a parfait with a carob-soymilk pudding sweetened with maple syrup bottom layer, and a fresh peach gelatin, sweetened with only apple juice and gelled with agar on the top. Everyone raved. They couldn't believe the gelatin "has seaweed in it". They were also astounded at how tasty "health foods" could be, but I told them I felt that term was ridiculous. "Shouldn't all foods be for health?" I asked. "What's everything else, then, disease food?" I went on about how our taste buds have become jaded over the years, and that if you give them a chance, simple grains, beans, vegetables, and fruits have an honest and satisfying flavor which people have become too desensitized to detect. Kathy sensed one of my familiar speeches coming on so she quickly changed the subject. She was right. There was no need for me to talk about the meal, since the food spoke for itself.

$$\boxed{\text{CHAPTER 22}}$$

BUTTERFLY DREAMS

It was a pleasantly warm June evening in 1990, a little humid, but not uncomfortably so. It was actually balmy with a light refreshing breeze that said rain would come soon. I was sitting outside with my four year-old daughter Sarah watching my seven year-old Elizabeth play Little League baseball. She and her teammates occupied one section of a schoolyard ball field, next to a large meadow.

At one point the breeze kicked up a little and a very strong, sweet, smell washed over us. It was dizzying. I looked over at the meadow and saw bush after bush of wild roses with their small white or pink flowers. After the game we walked over to get a closer look and smell, and found more - purple clover, honeysuckle, crown vetch, and other wildflowers I couldn't name. I told my girls to inhale deeply, and log it into their nose brains labeled "late Spring" so they'd never forget.

When the air is as moist as it was that evening, the smells seem to dissolve into the water particles and spread everywhere, as if they have been misted out of an atomizer. It was delicious. We saw our first butterfly of the season, too, working the meadow. At that moment, I wished I could be that butterfly, flitting from flower to flower, sucking up my fill of the intoxicating nectar.

The children were fascinated by butterflies, mystified by their transformations. They couldn't believe that the caterpillars we had seen lumbering around in the yard, eating huge holes in the wild cherry leaves, eventually changed themselves into the delicate creatures that don't so much fly, as float, balanced on moving air.

One of our favorite bedtime stories at the time was about a wise man who lived many years ago. One night he fell asleep and dreamed he was a butterfly. He floated on the breeze through a beautiful garden, stopping at each flower, uncoiling his spiral tongue, and drinking the sweet nectar. Then he awoke, but had a strange, disorienting feeling. He asked, "Am I a human being, now awake, who fell asleep and dreamed he was a butterfly? Or, am I a butterfly who was just awake, but is now asleep and dreaming he is a human being?"

Which world is real? Is the real world one of business lunches and dinner parties and wedding receptions and hands-in-the-snack-food-bag and fast-fat-food drive-throughs? Is it marbled meat conversations and dye on the plate and oil-soaked-wilted-whites that are supposed to be greens? Is it raped naked grains and artery-clogging goo? Is it a place where heart attacks and bypass surgery and breast cancer and colon cancer and hypertension and drugs drugs drugs drugs are accepted, inevitable, average, just the way things are?

And who are we? Are we fat and leaden and earth-bound, lumbering like caterpillars, only dreaming we can be butterflies? Or are we really those butterflies, now awake and floating, barely remembering the thread of a bad dream where we were heavy and stuck to the ground?

I think of these things whenever I move through a warm, moist June twilight, flitting from flower to flower, drunk on the smell and taste of purple clover and wild rose.

CHAPTER 23

EAT EIGHT GLASSES OF WATER A DAY

When patients confess that they don't do as well as they'd like with their diets, many are still proud that they drink plenty of water. No one has been able to tell me whether the advice came from a parent, a doctor, or a teacher, but I frequently hear that eight glasses a day is the magic number they need to cleanse their systems. I suspect that this is a relatively modern idea, probably only as recent as indoor plumbing, since it's hard to imagine a frontier person two or three hundred years ago making repeated trips to the stream with the old oaken bucket so that the family could all drink their daily 64 ounces of water.

Sometimes I'll ask the water-drinker, "Why do we need cleansing? What's so dirty?" Actually, we do generate a certain amount of bodily wastes which have to be eliminated. They are the breakdown products of the air we breathe, the food we eat, and other internal chemical reactions, and they have to be exhaled, sweated out, defecated and urinated away. Water is a vital part of all these removal processes, and a major component/vehicle of every type of waste, so it's true that we need to take in a certain amount to clean us out and keep the waste moving. I agree with the watery wisdom, but suggest we consider some other creative ways to do it.

Some foods naturally contain more water than others. Fruits and vegetables can be up to ninety percent water. Cooked whole grains and beans are mostly water, too. Meats and cheeses have very little water, and the advice to drink more water coincides with our modern tendency to make these foods central in our diets. We need to take in the extra water to make up for the water we're not getting from the foods in our diets, because we don't eat enough grains, beans, vegetables, and fruits. These animal-derived foods are more highly concentrated sources of protein (mostly from the animal's muscle). This protein generates a lot more nitrogen-containing waste products which have to be eliminated or else they will build up and poison us (ammonia is an example).

High carbohydrate foods such as the grains, beans, vegetables, and fruits tend to burn cleaner, breaking down ultimately into carbon dioxide and water. Both of these waste products are exhaled, while the latter also exits via sweat, urine, and bowel movements. These foods also contain some protein, especially the beans and grains, but it's less than in meat ounce for ounce and already comes packaged with water needed to eliminate it.

I think eight glasses of water a day is a good idea, but I'd prefer you get them off a dish instead. Eat watery foods, ones that either come with water naturally or foods to which you've added water. If you cook a cup of rice with a cup and a half of water, the water disappears when the rice is done. Where did it go? It's in the rice of course, and it goes into you when you eat it. It's the same with beans, barley, oatmeal - anything you cook with water. Those vegetables and fruits you water in your garden or the farmer waters in the field or the clouds water with rain soak up that liquid and carry it onto your dish. Start centering your diet around grains, beans, vegetables, and fruits, and amazing amounts of water will go into and come out of you, even though you're not drinking it directly from a glass. When I first restructured my way of eating I remember thinking, "Where's it all coming from?" Then I realized it was the watery food.

If you want to cleanse your system, do it with watery food which is intrinsically clean itself. Grains, beans, vegetables, and fruits can cleanse you because they already cleansed their own systems by drinking their own eight glasses of water. They drink it out of the earth or suck it out of your pot, then pass it on to you. Think of every spoonful of oatmeal, every forkful of broccoli, and every bite of an apple as a little serving of water in an unusual glass. Then drink heartily with your teeth.

CHAPTER 24

MIND YOUR T'S AND Q'S

I studied Macrobiotics for many years, a philosophy that came to this country from Japan and included specific dietary advice. One of my teachers, Michio Kushi, once told me that the founder and his teacher, George Ohsawa, used to enjoy eating cheesecake, even though this dessert would be anathema to anyone trying to eat a reasonably strict macrobiotic diet, since its major ingredients - dairy products and sugar - are proscribed. "Why did Ohsawa do it?" I asked. Kushi's answer was simple: "He liked it." When I asked how his system handled it, how he balanced the enormous load of fat and sugar, Kushi's told me that Ohsawa chewed each mouthful 350 times.

The Macrobiotic philosophy holds that thorough chewing can change the very nature of what you eat. They call it transmutation, an ability to transform something from bad to good. At first it didn't make sense to my Western-trained mind, because I couldn't see how all the chewing in the world could change fat and sugar into something else or make calories disappear. I could understand, though, that if you chewed a piece of cheesecake 350 times or even a hundred times, it would probably take quite a while to finish it. If the average piece of cheesecake can disappear in five bites and you allow two chews per second and one hundred chews per bite, it's over four minutes just to eat it, and that doesn't include the time between bites to talk, wipe your mouth with a napkin, sip tea, etc. So no matter how greasy and sweet the cheesecake is, if we chew long enough most of us probably won't have the time or desire to eat enough of it to affect us adversely.

After my right brain worked on Kushi's story about chewing and transmutation, I came up with the advice to mind your T's and Q's. The first T, Teeth, can affect another T, Time, since to chew thoroughly means you eat more slowly. Time, in turn, modifies the first Q, Quantity, since eating more slowly means you end up eating less. Quantity influences Quality, the second Q, since if you don't eat very much of something such as cheesecake or ice cream, it's less likely to hurt you.

You may occasionally find yourself in a situation where you have to or want to eat something you don't usually eat, something you feel wouldn't be very helpful if you ate it too often. Maybe it's a business lunch and you don't want to stand out or be considered too austere or less adventurous in front of an important client. Maybe it's a wedding reception or a dinner party and you don't want to insult the hosts. Don't worry. You shouldn't get hurt if you remember to chew as long and thoroughly as you can and mind your T's and Q's.

CHAPTER 25

QUICK START - 1992

Whenever I get to bed late, I usually pay for it the next day, since my internal alarm goes off at dawn regardless of the time I retire. I didn't fall asleep till after 2:00 am this morning, but for some reason my body clock gave me an extra thirty minutes today, so I'll have to hustle to get ready for work, and don't have time to prepare much of a breakfast. I'm so late I'll have to wrap up something and eat in the car. I don't like doing this and would rather be relaxing at the table, clearing out my head and preparing it for the day in those precious quiet moments of early morning. But I have to make compromises just as my patients tell me they do.

I know there's some whole wheat raisin bread around here somewhere. Two pieces go in the toaster, and while they are browning, I find some herbal tea still in the pot from last night, and I start it heating (it looks red, so it's probably something with rose hips). When the toast is done I quickly and irregularly spread on some apple butter, then pour in a little apple juice to sweeten the barely hot tea in my mug. It's bite chew chew, bite chew chew while driving, then sip sip sip at the traffic lights. I look around at other cars, and it seems that lots of folks are doing the same thing. Toast and a hot beverage is, after all, a pretty common breakfast, But the kind of bread, the kind of spread, and what's in the cup make all the difference, and can add a lot of value to this typical quick start.

I suspect that the people around me have something different in their napkins (something which stains them with oil, I'll bet), and something more jolting in their cups than I, but still I raise my mug to another commuter and nod my head, acknowledging our commonality. "Yes," my gesture says, "I'm one of you. We're all in this together."

As I think about it, it's just bread and water, but hardly prison fare. I think of it instead as the simple, stripped down building blocks for a human diet. There isn't a lot of fanfare or blaring noises. The day's work and pace will be enough to jolt me, so I don't need my breakfast to do it. I prefer this solo piano food to gently nudge me into my day. It doesn't stuff me either. After a bread and water breakfast, I don't need to send all my blood to my gastrointestinal tract, so I still have plenty left for my brain. And I still have plenty of hunger left in my bank account to drive me a few hours later in search of lunch.

$$\boxed{\text{CHAPTER 26}}$$

MANAGE YOUR TEAM

Joe is a thirty-eight year-old medical equipment salesman who has decided he needs to change his diet. He is mildly overweight (about twenty-five pounds), but otherwise apparently healthy. He has tried to lose weight several times before, usually on his own, but once his doctor referred him and his wife Melissa to a dietitian, they bought new cookbooks, and did it much more formally. Every time he has tried to lose weight he has succeeded, but only temporarily, as the weight always came back when he relaxed his regimen. This time he wants to fix it for good, because a recent serum cholesterol came back at a higher-than-average risk level of 225, and he knew a co-worker who was only 43 who'd had a heart attack and almost died fifteen months previously.

Joe thinks about going back to see the dietitian, but since he and Melissa already have the cookbooks and they've done it before, they decide to try it on their own again. They start with the four-ounce servings of skinless chicken, the pasta with meatless sauce, the salads with fat-free dressings, and the desserts of fresh fruit and fat-free frozen yogurt. He loses two pounds in the first month and feels frustrated because it seems to get harder every time, and he's uninspired by the meals.

Joe played baseball in high school and college and currently belongs to two softball teams, and coaches nine year-olds in a local

Little League. In the autumn and winter he plays basketball twice a week. He can't understand how he can be as active as he is and still not lose weight, especially since he claims, "I really don't eat that much."

Joe, let's try something new. Let's use your love and knowledge of baseball to fix your diet for good.

Imagine that all the foods in your diet are like the players on a professional baseball team and you are the manager. You arrive at spring training, that transition period between the off-season and the on-season, the same way you have arrived at that point in your life where you are abandoning the on-off diets you followed before and are ready to make a permanent change. You have a large number and variety of players, and your job is to find fifteen or so who will win the most games for you and form your regular starting lineup and pitching rotation. You will assign the rest of the players various supporting roles - relief pitchers, pinch-hitters, late inning defensive specialists, or to assume more prominent positions when a regular is injured or tired. Similarly, Nature and human know-how have provided you with a variety of foods—some basic and nourishing, and some more playful. Your job is to put them in order, to manage your food-team, to get a core of primary foods around which you center your diet, then assign the other foods various supporting roles.

Based on their past performances for you or other managers, or what you have heard about them from the scouts who read diet-books or listen to talk-shows, whole grains, beans and legumes, and fresh vegetables and fruits will probably be your starters. Animal-derived foods such as lean meats and low fat dairy products can pinch hit or relief pitch a few times a week, and maybe even start a game or two. Chocolate mousse and ice cream will usually sit on the bench, because if you let them play regularly you will probably have a losing season. Once in a while, though, a taste of one or the other can give the team a lift, so feel free to let them see action on special occasions when the team is so far ahead in a particular game that the outcome is not in question (such as when your weight is stable and where you want it, your blood pressure or blood sugar is under control, and your cholesterol is in the low risk category).

There's a lot of trial and error at first, but that's what spring training is all about. It's a time to work out the bugs, to get the machine running smoothly. In your new way of eating you will learn from experience which foods and meals taste and work best. Brown rice may be your whole grain of choice, or you may prefer barley or whole grain bread. You may like lentils more than chickpeas, and broccoli instead of cabbage. Every food gets a chance to show what it can do, and the ones which demonstrate superior talent and endurance will get to play most often. Others will better at short bursts and get spot-duty, become the part-time players, such as fish or chicken or low fat cheese.

Before you know it the season begins and it's time to get down to the business of winning ball games. No matter how much talent you have on the team and how well you have assigned players to their various roles, you can't just turn them loose on the field and let them play. You still have a lot of managing to do, because winning often depends on difficult judgment calls. Sometimes you play conservatively, strictly by the percentages - always letting a left-handed batter face a right-handed pitcher, always sacrificing the runner from first base to second with a bunt. Other times you are more daring - an unexpected hit-and-run, a suicide squeeze, walking the bases loaded to get the potential out at any base, having your third baseman charge the plate on a suspected bunt.

You'll get the most out of your regular players if you let them play almost every day. They will stay sharp and on their games if they see a lot of action. Always be on guard, though, because they can get tired, too, so know when you need to rest them a day or two. It's a long season and a long life, and these foods have to see you through to the end. If you've eaten brown rice five days in a row then substitute pasta or whole grain bread or couscous or tortillas or corn for a game or two. That's why you've got the large roster. Or if you've had whole grains every night for two weeks and now you're at a restaurant or a dinner party and all they've got is white rice or white bread or white noodles and you decide to eat nothing, don't be silly. It's only one night. Or at that same restaurant if the dessert tray looks very appealing but you usually play a whole-grain-crusted-fresh-fruit-juice-sweetened cobbler in that role, relax. One serving of their eggy-sugary carrot cake isn't going to kill you.

Some days it seems to go so easily: your lead-off hitters get on base with singles or by working-the-walk, then the meat of your line-up, the power hitters bring them home with doubles, triples, and home-runs, just the way it's supposed to work. On those days your team seems to be in a groove, and scoring seems effortless. The diet groove is similar: you're eating very simple foods but the meals are satisfying and your weight and cholesterol levels drop even though you're eating a lot.

On other days it seems that everyone is running in quicksand and you have to scrounge and scrape for every run you get: an infield hit on a close play at first that the other manager argues with the umpire, a stolen base after six or seven pick-off attempts, and finally a couple of sacrifice ground or fly balls just to get one, measly, it-will-never-be-enough run. Or else you make all the right decisions by the book but nothing seems to go your way and you can't score at all. Your players hit the ball solidly and hard, but right into the gloves of the opposing players, or just miss the holes and gaps between defenders, or you're foiled by bad hops or their center-fielder's spectacular catch against the wall to end your potentially big inning with runners stranded on first and third. It's the same way when the vegetables taste bland, or the rice is too mushy, or the dry whole wheat toast cries out for butter, but despite all this austerity you only drop a pound in two weeks. Don't worry, though. Feel confident that you put together a good team and stick to your original strategy and soon the base hits will start dropping and so will the pounds.

So loosen up. Don't be afraid to enjoy yourself. Be careful when you must, but be daring once in a while, too.

Okay. Enough talk. Time to play ball.

CHAPTER 27

GUIDED BY TEETH

When I studied anatomy and physiology in medical school I learned about the relationship between structure and function. Body parts are built or have developed a certain way to facilitate a certain function which gives or at some point gave the animal or plant some evolutionary or biological advantage. If a structure doesn't serve some function, theoretically it will eventually die off by means of natural selection. If a structure doesn't favor survival, the plant or animal which carries the trait for that characteristic won't live long enough to pass it on to offspring.

About eighteen years ago, I learned something about the structure and function of teeth from Macrobiotic teacher Michio Kushi. Ever wonder why we have teeth? Obviously they are there to process our food, to get it small enough to swallow and digest. But why do we have the specific *kinds* of teeth we have, the four canines, the eight incisors, and the twenty molars? Mr. Kushi says they tell us what we should be eating, because every different tooth is built to do a different thing, to handle a different kind of food.

Let's start with the canines. We have four of these - two top and two bottom, just to the outside of the four front teeth (the incisors). As the name suggests, canines are like dog teeth - pointed. Actually they resemble the teeth of any carnivorous animal, and are designed for ripping or tearing flesh (not very pretty, but that's what they do).

A serrated steak knife is like a long row of canine teeth. Kushi says that the fact that only four out of our thirty-two teeth are canines (a 1 to 8 ratio) suggests that flesh foods should only comprise one-eighth of our diet and that if we were supposed to eat more meat, we'd have more pointed teeth.

Next come the incisors, our front teeth. There are eight of these, and they are broad and flat. Incise means to cut, as in the word incision, but I think of these teeth more as choppers. They remind me of the big cleaver I use to chop vegetables and fruits. They make such nice cuts through stems, roots, and leaves, so that if you chew long enough, you will actually dice what is in your mouth. By the numbers, eight incisors out of thirty-two teeth implies that two parts out of every eight or one-quarter of everything we eat should be vegetables and fruits.

Finally we have our twenty molars - ten top and ten bottom - like short columns with small ridges or points on the surface. Finding the appropriate tool analogy is a little more difficult, because people rarely do in their kitchens what these teeth do, nor do they commonly see it done commercially. These teeth are grinders. Years ago, if you wanted to convert a grain or other seed into a flour for breads you would either have to grind it at home or have it ground for you at a local mill. The grindstones or millstones look something like molars - short columns of stone with small ridges that crush the grains between them. These teeth are similarly best suited for crushing and grinding seed foods such as grains and beans. It's like turning them into flour inside your mouth. Twenty molars suggests that five-eighths of our diet should be grains, beans, and other crushable seed foods

When I first read Kushi's rationale, it sounded too fanciful, and my left brain put together some counter-arguments. I speculated that we only need four canines because these teeth work so efficiently. Besides, meat doesn't need as much processing in the mouth, because stomach acid and pancreatic enzymes do most of the digestive work as opposed to teeth and salivary enzymes. I created my own structure-function explanation for the shape of the incisors, saying that they needed to be flat so the tongue could form the consonants d, t, z, and the diphthong th.

Then my right brain intervened and told me not to take it so literally. Now I look at the teeth as another cue, not as the orthodox interpretation of their structural significance. The relative proportions of foods suggested by dental shapes make sense anyway since they conform to what's on the Department of Agriculture's pyramid. But I'm always after something simpler, something I can remember without consulting a book, video, or nutritionist. When I use my teeth as a diet guide, I carry the information with me all the time, and knowing what to eat is as simple as opening my mouth and counting. It's thirty-two diet lessons planted in my gums.

CHAPTER 28

BRUSH THE TEETH DOOR SHUT

I remember when dental hygiene was a lot less complicated, when the only thing you had to do for your teeth at home was brush after eating and, of course, avoid between meal treats. It was so simple. Some time after that, in my teens I think, flossing was added, which increased the maintenance time significantly. Now it seems that every time I visit the dental hygienist I find out about more tools and more procedures: tiny-bristle brushes to get between the teeth (I thought the floss took care of that area), rubber-tipped gum-stimulators, little plaque-scraping hooks, and a vast array of spraying, vibrating, and polishing appliances.

I'll say one thing for the newer, more complicated, more time-consuming home dental care - after I brush, do a couple of laps around the uppers and lowers with the floss, tiny brush, and scraper, I don't want to eat again any time soon. It's just too much trouble to go through the whole routine again. Once I complete my nightly tooth trip, I'm definitely done eating until the next day, so I put a sign on my teeth that says *Closed Until Morning.*

Many people get into trouble eating after dinner (excluding those people with medical problems who require late-night snacks, such as insulin-requiring diabetics or folks with certain stomach or esophageal problems). Eating at night when you're less likely to be physically active and burn off what you ate may provide you with excess fuel which ends up stored around the abdomen or on the hips and thighs. In a 1993 article in the magazine *Hippocrates*, Japanese Sumo wrestlers claim that going to sleep after a large meal is one of the key strategies they use to attain their considerable weights (the author, Mary Roach, suggests that anyone who wants to lose weight should do the opposite).

Brushing your teeth brings eating to closure for the day. Once that clean, fresh taste is in the mouth, it's a disincentive to contaminate it again with food. But brushing the teeth alone isn't enough for me, because it's too quick and easy to simply brush them again if I eat again. But if I follow the brush with all the other tools, it's a different story. Once a night is enough.

So if I can't get people to eat more sensibly, perhaps I can get them to eat less by complicating their dental routines. Make the last course at dinner a loaded toothbrush, then brush, floss, and scrape till the teeth doors are shut.

$$\boxed{\text{CHAPTER 29}}$$

COLONIAL CHICKEN - 1995

Our friends Neil and Lynne had suggested we visit Colonial Williamsburg at Christmas time. They talked about the enchantment of candle-lit windows in eighteenth-century homes, all evergreen-bedecked, and moonlit lantern walking tours. Kathy and I were in the mood for a transporting experience, something to temporarily lift us out of our everyday world of the five-day grind, homework, and basketball practice, so we picked a three-day weekend in early December and drove down with Elizabeth and Sarah. Just before we arrived an Arctic air mass had crashed into a low pressure system coming up from the Gulf of Mexico and coated the whole area with snow. It was unusual for that time of year in southern Virginia, but lovely.

People who know me and also know Colonial Williamsburg said, "You won't find much to eat down there." People commonly tell me things like that, and I always find myself surprised because, while I was fairly rigid with my diet seventeen or eighteen years ago, I see myself as significantly relaxed these days. I eat some poultry now and then, accept white bread and white pasta when whole grain isn't available (something I would have never done before), and even take tastes of *real* desserts here and there. I suppose that what's relaxed for me still appears pretty austere to most other people.

We lodged in Williamsburg's restored area, so we could walk everywhere we had to go, even to supper at one of the colonial taverns on Saturday night. It was cold. We had layers of shirts and sweaters and thermal undies and boots and gloves and wool hats and it still felt very cold. We obviously weren't acclimated yet, but as Garrison Keillor once said after a surprise blizzard in Minnesota, those of us who felt we weren't ready for winter found out that winter was ready for us.

Duke of Gloucester Street, the main drag in town, was dark, except for occasional wire-baskets-of-fire hanging from eight-foot poles which served as streetlights. Outside each of the three taverns was a large bonfire where waiting patrons could warm themselves and watch the sparks jump, spin, and float off to nothing in the black sky. The children noticed the obvious similarity to summer fireflies, and had a little epiphany as they realized how those insects got their name. Even though we only spent a brief time outdoors, I was hungry for something to warm me, to help me adapt to this late-autumn/early winter weather. Let's just say I wasn't hankering for alfalfa sprouts and cold cucumber soup, but wanted something hot and heavy.

The tavern was absolutely charming. We sat next to a somewhat distressed brick wall, read the menu by candlelight, and listened to a white-stocking-ed, knickerbocker-ed, waist-coat-ed waiter tell us about the evening's specials. I commonly order seafood when I eat out at an American restaurant (that is, anything that isn't a rice and vegetable Oriental, a beans and cornmeal Mexican, a pasta primavera olive oil Italian, or a new-age/nouveau cuisine/black bean sauce/lite fare/stir-fry/up scale/yup scale place), because it's usually the only thing I can get fairly plain, with salad and baked potato and make a decent meal out of it while still looking and acting as if I'm one-of-the-gang. But the "Fish-of-the-day was salmon, which somehow didn't seem quite right after looking at tri-corner hats and watching/listening to the clomp-click-clomp of horse-drawn carriages all day. I wanted something Williamsburg-y, something with a look and sound and flavor that fit the flavor of the place and time. Then my eye caught and locked onto something which looked, on paper, to be exactly what I wanted - Barnyard, Spit-Roasted Chicken.

I've always felt that a good story makes a food or a meal come alive, and maybe even more nourishing in some transcendent, new-agey way. When I read the words *Barnyard* and *Spit-Roasted*, I immediately conjured up the image of a December colonial farm: there were a few cows, sheep, and a pig or two inside a split-rail fence. The pigs had their own pen, of course, while the cows and sheep were grazing on stiff, short, sparse brown grass. A kitchen garden sat a little closer to the house, long dead except for a couple of hardy cabbages. Eight or nine chickens pecked around for a stray seed or a dried worm (these were free-ranging chickens before there was anything besides free-ranging for contrast).

A woman entered the scene, wearing a white duster cap and a long linen skirt, bundled in a linsey-woolsey shawl. The animals didn't pay much attention until she bent over to grab one of the birds, which scattered the others, as if they knew what was going on. After the bloody ritual from which most of us are conveniently insulated, she took the chicken inside a dark kitchen, plucked it, dressed it, then let it roast on a spit inside the huge, walk-in fireplace. It would be warm and satisfying for her husband and children who had worked outside all day, hands numb as they split wood or repaired the barn or wagon.

I realize I am seriously deluded. I never saw anyone in Williamsburg scooping up any barnyard chickens, so I'm sure the birds are truck-delivered by the hundreds, already plucked and gutted by a local processing plant. And even though I didn't actually see the tavern's kitchen, I have to believe that a restaurant in a major American tourist area serving several hundred people a night has the most modern cooking equipment available, rather than the cozy hearth I imagined. But my way is a lot more fun, and I swear the meal was tastier and more digestible because of my little fantasy.

As you can probably tell by now, I eat very little meat. I usually don't care much for the taste or the texture, and most times I'm not crazy about the whole idea. When we first sat down and I scanned the menu, I thought I'd have a disappointing meal, except for the surprise whole wheat rolls and some salad. But I have to tell you that my Barnyard, Spit-Roasted Chicken was righteous. Phrases such as "the meat practically fell off the bone" and "it melted in my mouth" are clichés, but now I know their origin. Now I can relate.

After dinner I was ready to brave the cold fire-lit night again. I was ready to pick up a musket and join the Continental Army. I was ready to go back to our room and slip into sweet chair-sleep as my children watched re-runs of 70's sitcoms, all warm and dreamy and satisfied.

CHAPTER 30

PLATE IT, TABLE IT, AND EAT IT OFF YOUR FEET

What do you do when it's 11:30 pm and your hand is deep inside a 10-ounce potato chip bag? This is Joanne's recurrent dilemma. She's a forty-six year-old overweight diabetic Nursing Assistant who works the 3 pm to 11 pm shift in a Nursing Home. She says she feels "keyed up" when she gets home which makes her hungry, and finds that a snack relaxes her. She knows that it's a bad idea because she goes to sleep within half an hour so "it probably all turns to fat." She can go through half a bag in five to ten minutes. "I just shovel them in," she says, "four or five at a time," standing at her kitchen counter looking through the mail. That half-bag represents about 700 calories, almost 500 coming from fat. If she did it every day she'd gain six pounds every month.

For a while she stopped buying the chips, then started picking them up for her husband and children. "Why should I deny them?" she asked, "they don't have a weight problem or diabetes." She also tried substituting low fat pretzels or lower calorie baked chips, but found herself eating a larger quantity because she thought they were safer.

I've already provided several solutions for Joanne throughout this book. She could summon her border guard to read the nutrition label on the potato chip bag and let her know that the 1400 calories in the whole bag is a lot of energy which she didn't pre-burn scrubbing and slicing potatoes or mashing corn and cotton seeds to extract the oil. This could buy her some time while she starts to relax and possibly stop the chain reaction that began when she walked into the kitchen and up to the cabinet. She could unmask what she thought was hunger and identify her emotions as the cause of her "keyed up" feeling, not really hunger. At the same time she could realize that she had eaten ate dinner only four hours earlier, and didn't expend a whole lot of energy afterwards (the Nursing Home gets pretty quiet after 9 pm when there's no bathing, dressing, or transferring in and out of chairs since most of the residents are in bed by then). On days she doesn't work she eats supper around 6 pm and doesn't need to eat half a bag of potato chips before bed.

Now here's another technique she can use. If she really wants a snack and it has to be potato chips, she should plate it, table it, and eat it off her feet. She should count out ten chips which represents about 100 - 110 calories, place them on a small plate or even in a tea cup where they would stack higher and look like more, then close the bag and put it away. She should put the dish or cup on a table, then sit down and eat them slowly, one-half to one chip at a time. When the plate is clean or the cup is empty, the snack is over. The plate is crucial to define the portion, or else the whole bag or box may become the serving size. The instruction to sit at the table is just as important, since it frames the event, gives it a definite beginning and end. Standing to eat is more open-ended, since you can keep moving around –to get the mail, hang up a coat, listen to phone messages – and be eating the whole time.

The other nice thing about this technique is that it avoids any sense of deprivation. I didn't say, "Don't eat it", but "if you're going to eat it, do it this way". She could still have what she wanted, as long as she changed the way she got it. It's like using a new frame to give an old picture a completely different look.

Humans aren't cars that need their fuel tanks filled at the end of a long ride. We aren't horses, either, and don't need a feed-bag strapped on at the end of work day. The advice to plate it, table it, and eat it off your feet is more than a clever behavioral cue, but a way to add dignity and reverence to a common but nonetheless sacred act.

Melody

CHAPTER 31

SLOGANS

I believe that the pervasive and persuasive influence of advertising is one of the reasons the patients I see consume too much of the wrong stuff and for the wrong reasons. I detect a seductive appeal about eating a certain fast food or drinking a certain soft or hard drink, a belief that it will somehow make life more like it is in the commercial - more fun, more interesting, and overall just better. Unfortunately, the reality often falls far short of the created expectation, at which point a disappointed consumer could rightfully say, "Hey! What gives? I drank the stuff, so where's the beach, the volleyball game, and the girls?" If these ads wanted to be more honest, I would suggest they show these beer-guzzling and hamburger-chomping people years later - in cardiac care units after heart attacks, or getting their chemotherapy treatments.

The advertising slogans, in particular, strike me as catchy little bytes which are easy to remember and associate with a particular product. Over the years I heard that a soft drink tastes like love or that milk is a natural and beef builds strength. Simple wholesome foods, however, have been under-represented, so I think it's time to balance the scales and develop slogans for some of the foods I've talked about in this book. I won't use beach scenes or skimpy short pants to sell this stuff, since I assume you are all intelligent enough to respond to a simpler message.

Let's start with whole grains and beans. We can play on the fact that these foods are actually the seeds of cereal grasses and leguminous vines which, if planted, would sprout and grow.

Whole grains and beans: where new life begins, for plants AND you.

Or how about this take-off from a recent national campaign for a car the manufacturer and their ad agency wanted us to think was "what to drive".

Whole grains and beans: what to eat.

Here are a couple for vegetables.

Root vegetables: they go deep for life so they can bring life to you.

The importance of something as simple and familiar as carrots and the role Vitamin A plays in vision might be remembered this way.

Carrots are busy making carotene in the dark so you can see the light.

I might advertise the sun-trapping, photosynthetic power of green leafy vegetables this way.

Catch some rays the safe way: eat leafy greens.

Or how about this one: *Sunshine without the burn: leafy greens.*

I could create some excitement about the recently discovered benefits of the indoles and isothiocyanates in cruciferous vegetables this way.

Peter Rabbit was onto something: check out the cabbage patch.

For fruits, perhaps I would resurrect the image of Mother Nature I used earlier.

Fruit: sweetness the way Mother intended or
Fruits come sweet and colored: no need to add a thing.

For meats, dairy foods, salt, sweeteners, fats, and oils, two short phrases say it all: *Highly concentrated, a little goes a long way.*

Finally, for anything heavily chemicalized or artificially manipulated, conjure up the image of Mother Nature one more time:

If Mother doesn't recognize it, it probably isn't food.

$$\boxed{\text{CHAPTER 32}}$$

BLIZZARD OF '96

It's been seventeen years since the Blizzard of '79, and a lot has changed. Now I work in an office where appointments can be canceled and rescheduled when two and a half feet of snow fall, as they did here on January 7th and 8th, 1996. There are no anxious waits by the telephone operator's window, straining to see the car of my night-shift relief, and no long fruitless treks to empty trolley stops or deserted highways. I didn't need to hitch a ride with a rear-wheel-drive madman, out looking for a sale in the middle of a paralyzing winter storm. Instead, I was home and safe and moved several tons of snow off of a driveway and walkways with a single aluminum bent-handle shovel in six back-breaking, elbow-straining shifts.

What doesn't changed, though, is dinner. I still walked inside with the sweat crystallizing on my wool cap to the wonderful aroma of split pea soup and brown rice. It tasted just as holy, went down just as easily, and was every bit as satisfying as it had been in 1979. After two bowls of each, I pushed myself away from the table, and in a bold move declared this my official blizzard meal.

CHAPTER 33

MY FAVORITE MEAL - TODAY

My favorite meal is the one I am eating and need right now. It's the one I imagined coming home from work, then found with patient, genuine hunger after hurdling over unmasked boredom and frustration. I started to digest it while I was still only smelling it, and it started to heal me before a morsel ever crossed my border-mouth.

It's the meal that has all the plant parts - roots, leaves, fruits, and seeds on which I spend my precious appetite. I fashioned it from love and respect, not rules or fear, and it contains my labor and sweat, and the labor and sweat of countless others I thank with head-bowed grace. It's the meal Mother Nature would recognize and embrace as her own, and the one that shows animals, barely, if at all, buried under leaves. It moves me forward along the caterpillar-butterfly continuum.

It's a meal made by a goose-brain who knows when to honk and when to fly south, away from death, and it goes down like water when I finish chewing. I eat it off a plate, off a table, and off my feet, and my grandmother might have cooked the same thing. It's the meal I composed, arranged, and conducted into the music that takes me home.

CHAPTER 34

MY DIET HOME

Remember Dorothy Gale? She was harassed by Miss Gulch. Uncle Henry and Auntie Em were so busy with the farm they didn't have time for her and her seemingly unimportant concerns about a dog. She dreamed of a land "somewhere over the rainbow... where troubles melt like lemon drops". Then the cyclone blew in, she got a major bump on the head, and dreamed she had actually twisted her way to that place on the other side of the colored arch.

Unfortunately, Dorothy's troubles didn't melt so easily in the land of Oz. She had about as much as she could handle with the Wicked Witch of the West. Sure, it all very colorful, with green horses and yellow brick roads, and there were lots of adventures. But when all was said and done, all she really wanted to do was get back to Kansas, to get back home. With a little help from her friends, she eliminated the witch ("liquidated her" as the Wizard put it), and brought the charred broomstick to the great and powerful Oz so he could keep his promise and grant her wish - to go back home. Just when it seemed the Wizard was going to renege on his promise, Dorothy's dog, Toto, pulled back a curtain and exposed Oz as just an ordinary man working some pretty fancy machinery. He was nothing more than a glib Midwest state fair showman who had wandered into Oz in his hot air balloon on a prevailing wind. After the truth was out, the Wizard promised to take her home personally in his balloon;

unfortunately, he took off accidentally without her. She yelled, "Come back!" but the airborne Oz shouted back, "I can't! I don't know how it works." So much for wizardry.

Just when she thought she'd be stuck in Oz forever, Dorothy's guardian angel, good witch Glynda bubbles onto the scene and tells her she had always had the power to get home - the ruby slippers. All she had to do was click her heels and say, "There's no place like home." First, though, Glynda wants to know whether or not the young girl has learned anything. Dorothy summarizes it this way: "The next time I go looking for the other side of the rainbow, I won't look any further than my own back yard. If it isn't there, I never lost it to begin with." Which means, I think, that if it isn't in your own back yard, you never had it in the first place. Here's an even looser interpretation: if it isn't in your own back yard, it isn't anywhere.

I talk to people every week who search today for the dietary equivalent of the land over the rainbow. They look for quick fixes that will melt pounds the way Dorothy wanted her troubles to melt, as when Rita asked me if Chromium Picolinate would help her lose weight. They look for dietary magic bullets in the foreign and exotic, believing it has to come from some thing or some one outside their own experience, and often ignore the common, familiar magic all around them all the time. People tell me that they take pulverized barley grass from Japan, ginseng root from Korea, special water from European springs, tea from the bark of a Brazilian tree, algae from a pristine lake in Oregon or Hawaii, or oils from Arctic fish. There's nothing wrong with any of these practices, which are fun, adventuresome, and somewhat titillating. But I tell my patients they're doing themselves a disservice if they believe their lives and good health depend on these substances, and get distracted from the wonders waiting right in their own back yards.

I decided to look figuratively in my own backyard and examine the eating habits and patterns of my genetic and geographic grandparents – the people I came from, and the people who came from where I live.

Post-colonial America is a nation of immigrants. While Native Americans might be able to trace their ancestors back thousands of years or across the Bering Sea, everyone else is connected to someone born in Europe, Africa, or Asia going back only several hundred years at most, and in many cases considerably less. This means that my genetic and geographic grandparents lived in very different places and ate very different kinds of foods. Because modern food production and transportation have homogenized our dietary habits to a large extent (people can get the same hamburger and frozen peas in Philadelphia they can in San Francisco), it may be hard to remember that the way people used to eat was determined by what they could grow or hunt *where they lived*. This means that there were no oranges to garnish the first Thanksgiving Day feast, and no bananas in the cornucopia.

My ancestry is southern European-Mediterranean. My mother's parents were born in Italy, and my father's in Sicily. My surname is French, but since Sicily is an island, peoples from throughout the Mediterranean and even from further north visited and settled there, hence Greek ruins, redheads, and other seeming anomalies. My geographic grandparents were the Lenni-Lenape Indians of southeastern Pennsylvania who farmed in addition to hunting and gathering in the local fields and woodlands. Given these two sets of grandparents, maybe I am supposed to eat cornmeal mush sprinkled with Parmesan cheese, along with Jerusalem artichokes, violet leaf salad, and wild grouse sautéed in garlic and olive oil with a chickpea-pinto bean sauce. You're all invited over for melting pot luck. I'm talking here about a way of eating based not so much on nutrition texts or popular diet books or talk shows, but arising out of genes and geography, blood and soil.

The Lenni-Lenape and Delaware Indians who lived in my area called their main foods the *three sisters* - corn, beans, and squash. These foods all grew very well together, something we'd call companion planting today. The corn stalk grew straight and tall, the bean vines twisted and curled around the stalk, and the squash/pumpkin plants spread on the ground all around the corn and beans. One of the local Lenni-Lenape bands was the *Okehocking*, which comes from a word meaning people of the pumpkin place Corn, however, was the staple, as it was for so many Native Americans. When I drive along the road in October and see decorations made from colored corn, pumpkins, and gourds, it strikes me that we use these as symbols and adornments, while our geographic ancestors depended on them for sacred sustenance.

In addition to the three sisters, the local Indians ate a wide variety of local vegetables, fruits, nuts, seeds, and of course, game. Many native Americans foods grow literally in my back yard: wild carrots (white roots that actually taste more like parsnip); dandelions (edible leaves and roots, and flowers often used to make wine); violet leaves; curly dock; lamb's quarters; nettles; black walnuts; black cherry; wild mustard; wild garlic; and many others. I once read an article in *Sports Illustrated* about wild foods foraging in which the author said that if the Jolly green Giant hadn't domesticated it, then it probably wasn't any good. I disagree, since one person's weed is another one's feast.

But it goes beyond taste. For me, it's also about feeling connected. I have a cookbook entitled *Native Harvests: Recipes and Botanicals of the American Indian* by Barrie Kavasch which has a recipe for pumpkin black walnut soup. I decided to try making it a few years back, happy to have some use for the million or so black walnuts that fall into my yard every late summer-early autumn, often dropping like bombs while I rake leaves. Trying to get them open, though, is another matter. After breaking my nutcracker and denting my boot heel, I finally resorted to a sledgehammer. This worked, but it was still another five or ten minutes per nut to dig out the meat. The Lenni-Lenape must have had a better system, or would have otherwise starved. It was worth the work, though, since the walnuts have a deliciously rich taste. I used a pumpkin from my garden, and added the small amount of maple syrup specified in the recipe. I hadn't made the syrup, but pretended I had, and felt justified doing so because I had made some from sap several years earlier. Eating the soup was a religious experience for me. Besides providing me with a labor-intense calorie pre-burning autumn afternoon project and adding some flavor and nourishment to my diet that day, the simple meal grounded me. It made me feel that I belonged somewhere and could walk a few yards to find all I would ever need.

My mother's mother was born in central Italy, near Naples, around the turn of the century. She came to this country at eleven with her older brother. What courageous people. At the same age I was barely crossing the street by myself, let alone the Atlantic Ocean on a crowded ship, a stranger coming to a strange land. Like so many other immigrants, they were able to assimilate the new while still retaining much of the old.

A few years after her husband died my grandmother came to live with our family when I was eight or nine years old. She helped my mother with various household chores, including the cooking. I remember my grandmother's spaghetti sauce being very light and thin. At that same time, television commercials usually pictured very thick, rich sauce, covering the pasta like lava. Grandmom told us never to drink water with our meals, or else our stomachs would swell and hurt. She made her own pizza dough from scratch, rolling it out with a well-seasoned broom handle (before they started painting them). I can still see the ceramic bowl with a towel on top, in which the yeasty mound would rise. In addition to the well-known tomato and cheese pie, she often put vegetables on top, such as spinach or broccoli, which restaurants do these days as well. One thing I've never seen in a restaurant, though, is raisins, which she put on the pizza with spinach. The sweetness of the dried fruit and the bitterness of the greens on a home-made crust with just the right amount of olive oil and garlic is something I can savor even as I write about it, something that tastes even better with the distortion of time, the haziness of memory.

Lentil soup was a Friday night staple in winter (as Catholics, we avoided meat in those days). I admit I wasn't crazy about it at the time, but I ate it. I eat a lot of it now, and always think of my grandmother when I do. I can still see her sitting at the kitchen table, eating a lunch that consisted only of some sautéed dandelion greens which she mopped up with the hard end of a loaf of crusty bread.

"Grandmom," I would say, "is that all you're gonna eat?" (meaning no hamburger, no luncheon meat) "That's all I want," she would say.

She worked very hard, dusting and sweeping and cooking literally until two days before she died. She brought her rosary beads to Mass. She cried when President Kennedy was shot, and was saddened when Pope Paul VI needed a protective bubble top on his limo in a New York City parade. Kennedy's assassination had been hard enough to accept, but it was inconceivable to her that anyone would try to shoot the pope. She ate a lot of grains, vegetables, and beans. She ate very little overall, and very little else.

My father's father grew up on a small farm on a hill near Messina in Sicily. His family was very poor. Their house, little more than a shack, had no plumbing or electricity. Years later, when my father went back to visit the place, the house was still standing. He was amazed and shocked at how primitive it was. When he returned he asked his father how he could ever live in such a place. Grandpop was cool. He said, "Why do you think I left for America?" Good answer.

He did leave for America, in the same wave of immigrants that brought my mother's mother and so many others. The only time he ever returned to Europe was to fight for the Allies in World War I. Perhaps fight is the wrong word and represent might be more appropriate, since he told us he sat in a front line trench and never fired a shot. "They never did anything to me," he said.

He came to Philadelphia at a time when people got around by foot and trolley, and he continued to walk everywhere even into his 90's. He made his own wine and, during Prohibition, his own beer too. Wedged into the mirror frame in his dining room was a small picture of Saint Anthony of Padua, patron saint of lost things. I asked him once about life in the old country. He remembered it well, despite leaving so young. He remembered being so poor that he and his brothers would take off their shoes to walk down the mountain since they didn't want to wear out their shoes (I guess they were less concerned about wearing out their feet). I asked him about food, and he recalled growing or raising everything they needed on their small farm. They took their wheat into town to be milled into flour for pasta and bread. The bread was *pane' nero* - black bread. He didn't know it, but they were eating whole grain bread. Vegetables and fruits were abundant in the beneficent Mediterranean climate. They had their own olive trees, and pressed the fruit for oil.

"What about meat," I asked him, "didn't you ever eat meat?" "Sure," he said, and explained that there was always some chicken around. When I asked how often they ate red meat he said "Christmas and Easter." "Christmas and Easter," I said, "was that all?" That was all. Amen.

He died at age ninety-two with all his own teeth. I don't know for sure if his way of eating helped him live so long so well. I don't know if exercise which wasn't exercise at the time but simply transportation and food production and dancing helped him live so long so well. I don't know if an attitude which balanced acceptance (if you want me to go sit in a trench with a rifle and look at Germans, sure I'll go) with refusal to accept certain things (life has to better in America, so I'm leaving) helped him live so long so well. I don't know any of these things, but I believe them all.

I know I'm romanticizing, and I don't expect people to grow all their own food and make all their own pizza and maple syrup and pumpkin soup, and walk wherever they need to go, and forage for wild violet leaves and burdock roots, because I don't do all these things myself all the time. I only want us to eat more simply, as if we'd produced it ourselves, with knowledge of where it originated, and respect for the labor that brings it to us.

So I say thank you. To my genetic grandparents, for showing me the eating way home - the path that leads from the Old World to the New. I thank my parents for keeping it alive in stories, on faded, stained, and spotted 3 x 5 recipe cards, on the broom handle that has rolled out miles and miles of loving sustenance, and simmering on the stove.

I also thank my Indian grandparents of this place, my home. I feel our kinship when I walk through the fields and woods, looking at and sometimes picking or digging up the leaves, berries, and roots that you gathered. And when I eat these foods, our blood is the same, getting its life from this earth, my earth, our earth.

Okay, Dorothy. Get ready. It's time to do what Glynda said. I think we've learned what we had to learn, so let's tap our heels and go back to where we started. Sure it's colorful here in Oz, but it's a little crazy, too. Let's go back to the land of black and white, where our heads were clearer.

Tap them, Dorothy, and say it. With hearts and tongues, we say it too.

There's no place like home.
There's no place like home.
There's no place like home.

NOTES

Chapter 1

page 1   "Indiana Jones" refers of course to the character in the popular Steven Spielberg-George Lucas film *Raiders of the Lost Ark.*

Chapter 3

page 18   *The Desperate Hours* was a 1955 film directed by William Wyler, currently distributed by Malofilm Group.

Chapter 5

page 23   I was first introduced to Macrobiotics in 1979 through the small booklet *Macrobiotics: Experience the Miracle of Life*, taken from lectures by Michio Kushi, edited by Edward Esko, published in 1978 by East West Publications, a division of the East West Foundation. I learned more about this discipline in Mr. Kushi's *The Book of Macrobiotics*, from Japan Publications, Inc., 1977. I attended numerous lectures and seminars featuring Kushi and spent some time studying with him in Boston in the early 1980's.

Chapter 7

page 34   Information about the food pyramid frequently appears on food packaging, but is an official creation of the federal Department of Agriculture.

page 34   While the term "schematic plant" is mine, I believe that Macrobiotic teacher Michio Kushi may have first introduced me to the notion that eating grains, leafy greens, and root vegetables was something like eating an entire plant. It may have been at one of his lectures, since I couldn't find a specific reference in my collection of his published work.

page 36   I first learned of the proposed connection between the "nightshade" plants and arthritis in *Nightshades and Health* by Norman F. Childers and Gerard M. Russo, Horticultural Publications, Somerset Press, Somerville, New Jersey, 1977.

Chapter 9

page 46   *Getting Well Again* was written by Dr. O. Carl Simonton with Stephanie Matthews-Simonton and James Creighton, published in 1978 by J.P. Tarcher, Los Angeles, and Bantam, New York in 1980.

Chapter 11

page 54   Pritikin Centers are residential lifestyle-modification facilities started by Nathan Pritikin, and now run by his son, Robert. The best known of these is in Santa Monica, California; I worked at the Downingtown, Pennsylvania location until it closed in October, 1989.

Chapter 12

page 57   Ruth Beebe Hill's *Hanta Yo* was published in 1979 by Doubleday & Company, Inc., Garden City, New York. The quote I use here is found on page 27.

Chapter 17

page 73   I recall the unsettling but simultaneously galvanizing image of death lurking over the left shoulder in several of Casteneda's books, but particularly in *Journey to Ixtlan*, Pocket Books, 1972.

Chapter 20

page 80   Paul A. W. Wallace's *Indians in Pennsylvania* was published in 1961 by the Pennsylvania Historical and Museum Commission.

page 80   *American Indian Myths and Legends* is a collection of stories edited by Richard Erdoes and Alfonso Ortiz, published in 1984 by Pantheon Books, New York.

page 80   A good description of how beef and dairy foods rose to their current prominent position in the American diet can be found in the 1981 Center for Science in the Public Interest book *Jack Sprat's Legacy* by Patricia Hausman.

page 84   See notes for Chapter 5 for the names of Kushi's Macrobiotic books.

Chapter 22

page 88   We encountered this story of the butterfly dreamer in the delightful book *Animalia* by Barbara Berger, published in 1982 by Celestial Arts, Berkley, California.

Chapters 24 & 27

pages 92,100   Refer to the note from Chapter 5 about Macrobiotics.

Chapter 28

page 104   *Hippocrates* is a monthly medical magazine published for physicians by Time Publishing Ventures, Inc., San Francisco, California. The article I refer to here was in the March, 1993, issue (Volume 7, Number 3), pages 50-60.

Chapter 29

page 106   The colonial taverns are owned and operated by the Colonial Williamsburg Foundation. The one I refer to in this chapter is Shields Tavern.

page 106   I heard Garrison Keillor say this one Saturday night on his popular public radio program *A Prairie Home Companion*.

Chapter 34

page 117   The 1939 MGM movie version of L. Frank Baum's *The Wizard of Oz* charmed me as a child and continues to captivate me. So full of metaphor and allegory, I still haven't completely plumbed its depths. The song *Over the Rainbow* was written by Harold Arlen with Lyrics by E.Y. Harburg.

page 119   Much of my information about local Native Americans came from *Edgmont: The Story of a Township*, published in 1976 by the author Jane Levis Carter, Edgmont Township, Pennsylvania.

page 120   I think I read the Sports Illustrated article in a dentist's office, or some other waiting room, and have no idea of the year, issue, or author's name.

page 120   *Native Harvests* was published in 1979 by Vintage Books, New York.